Happy Weight

Unlocking Body Confidence
Through Bioindividual Nutrition
and Mindfulness

D1445310

Danielle Della Valle, NTP

Bio + Well Nutrition
Vancouver, Washington

ISBN: 978-9986486-0-6

Bio + Well Nutrition books are available at special discounts when purchased in bulk for premiums and sales promotions as well as for fund-raising or educational use. Special editions or book excerpts can also be created to specification. For details, contact orders@happyweightbook.com.

Bio + Well Nutrition
www.biowellnutrition.com
Editing: Myles Aion, Lincoln Square Books
Cover design: Olivia Ashton Photography and Chloezola526 on Fiverr.com

I dedicate this book to all women who have ever felt as though they were unworthy of loving themselves or their bodies.

Acknowledgments

When I think about book dedications, I think about the standard molds and say to myself, wow, how can this fit every person's story? For me that would be impossible. It takes a village to make anything happen in life, and I would be lying if I said this book was just mine and maybe one other person's. I'll start by thanking my husband, Kenny. He is and will forever be the only person on this planet that actually gets me and gives me exactly what I need in this life. I am so grateful for his amazing ability to challenge me in every way possible and make me feel as though I can accomplish anything, if I put the work in.

Undoubted eternal thanks and gratitude to my mother and father, my number one fans, the two people who made me, literally. I am equal parts of their awesome and it shows. If I didn't have such unconditionally loving, passionate, colorful, and hardworking people as my parents, I would have never become the unique soul I am today.

Thanks also to my Nonie and Papa, the two most loving and supportive grandparents a woman could ever ask for. They always let me beat my own drum. I feel them with me every day and always seek to be close to them in the life I live even though they are no longer in this physical life. To my godmother, Kaaren, the woman that introduced me to nutrition and always made me feel comfortable as a child with natural inclinations to be a part of the holistic realm. To my amazing chosen family and to my actual family, thank you for never making me feel as though I was crazy or didn't belong in this world. You know who you are, thank you for loving me! Finally, to my instructor Cathy Eason who reminded me time and time again that there is no such thing as a one-size-fits-all approach, and that understanding the individual is the most important lesson one can learn.

To Melody Larue for being so brave and writing a very real and vulnerable chapter in this book about her journey to her Happy Weight, for her friendship, and kick ass personality!

To Kendall Kendrick my soul sister, for talking me off the ledge every time I was ready to give up.

To all of my amazing beta readers for giving me an honest opinion and being the first people to read the book! Ali Anderson, Beth Schultz, Elizabeth Bonne, and my amazing mother Shelley Brose', you all hold a very special place in my heart for making me feel like this was all worth it, I love you all so much!!!

I would also like to thank all of the editors that made this book what it is, Vinnie Kinsella for being the first person to ever read my manuscript in the early stages and to help me get the book on the right track. To Stephanie Gunning and Myles Aion for pushing my limits emotionally and intellectually and helping to make this book into this amazing final product. I couldn't have done it without you all!

To Olivia Ashton for your brilliance in photography, for being a sentient being of light and love, and making my book cover dreams come true! To any and every client I have ever worked with for sharing your deepest selves and allowing me to be a part of your story and mine, THANK YOU! And lastly to anyone who has supported me through this process, been a part of my story, and helped me to realize that I am doing this all for the greater good. I love you all!

Contents

INTRODUCTION
The History of Women and Beauty

Since the beginning of civilization, women have been concerned with appearance. The ancient Egyptians were one of the first civilizations in documented history that used tattoo makeup; they tattooed eyeliner and eyebrows on their faces to give them the appearance of beauty and to accentuate what was believed to be one of their most valued features. The women also shaved their heads to wear perfectly coiffed wigs, so that no hair was out of place. Vanity has always been a part of our culture, and modifying our physical features has been an obsession since we were conscious enough to understand that we had a face that we could change. If we look back into the historical timeline of beauty, we will find many ancient rituals still in use today. Tattooing was only the beginning, and other body modifications shortly followed. The Mayans would stretch their ears to fit stone plugs and, only adorned themselves with the finest stones they could find, like turquoise and jade. These stones were a sign of wealth and aristocracy. We forget historical expectations and believe that body image is a worry of our new era.

Today, women may suggest that Marilyn Monroe was the pinnacle of beauty and shape. Many women go as far as to claim that Marilyn Monroe wore a size 16. This couldn't be further from the truth. Marilyn Monroe in today's sizes would be a four, as she only weighed 118 pounds. So if you thought the 1950s and 1960s were a time where women were safe from ridicule, you would be gravely mistaken. Women have been objectified since the beginning of time. And let us not forget the clothing we have endured to "enhance" our beauty, like the corset. In the early 1820s, after the French Revolution, the corset was born. Sometime around the late 1820s the corset crossed the ocean and became a regular fashion piece in America. Women everywhere were eager to cinch and distort their waists to unnatural proportions. Unfortunately, the corset is still in play today. There are some celebrities, whom I have no interest in naming, who still use this tool to inspire women to a figure that is not only unnatural, but can be extremely harmful to internal organs.

We use so many undergarment devices to create the appearance of smooth lines, but for many of us, smooth lines are not realistic. For thousands of years we have been obsessed with changing the way we look, but for what? And for whom?

WHY ARE WE NOT ENOUGH?

Beauty is pain. I have been hearing this since I was young. I grew up in a southern California household knowing women who, quite frankly, hated their bodies; nothing was ever good enough. If it wasn't a facelift, it was Botox. If it wasn't Botox, it was trying to get back to their high school weight by any means necessary. Decreasing our calorie intake and starving ourselves is one way to say that we hate our body with a passion, and just want desperately to be thin.

What kind of message are we sending to the young girls around us? What kind of role model are we? Growing up in one of the plastic surgery capitals of the world did not make for a very secure personal image. Lucky for me, I left in my early twenties and moved to a more forward community that holds open conversations about health and well-being. But for the rest of the women in America, we may not be so lucky. The idea that to be beautiful, we must go through procedures or painful endeavors is obscene.

At the age of twenty-five, over 50 percent of my female friends had already undergone breast augmentation surgery. As far as I know, they hadn't considered the possible side effects or repercussions. Why were they not happy with the bodies they were born with? What made them feel incomplete? Why does society push us into undergoing major surgery to fix a mole? Why do we feel that we have to change our appearance to be happy and make others happy? And why do we continue to pass this idea down to the women we raise?

We should be lifting up the women in our community that we are responsible for, not putting them down.

How Do We Change?

The question is how, after millennia of needing to be something different from ourselves, do we make a change? How do we override the message in the billions of dollars worth of advertising we have seen that teach us to hate ourselves?

The answer is: We make the choice to do so. Every day that we wake up, we make a conscious choice of how we want to live our lives. Every day we make excuses and we continue living the same life simply because we are afraid to be different.

Trust me when I say I know how it feels to be on the receiving end of ridicule, of judgment, and disappointment. Pushing boundaries and stepping outside of the box separates us. It separates us from the people we think to be the bearers of truth, family members, friends, bosses, and parishioners. These people are so quick to push their opinions and ideas on us without asking. They give unsolicited advice and direction, whether or not it is not needed or wanted. It ends up confusing us, we don't know what choices to make, and they influence our decisions. The unfortunate aspect of this is that those people turn out to be just as confused as we are; because they are making it all up. Everyone is faking it in this life. Not one single person has all the answers. Have you ever heard the phrase "Fake it till you make it?" Most everyone is doing this. But it may still be scary to challenge those around us, and we might feel as though we will be left alone.

I want you to know that when you step outside the box, something beautiful happens: You become truly happy and fulfilled for the first time. In this book, my aim is to encourage you to take the risk to be yourself.

There is a community waiting for you to reveal yourself and be who you genuinely are. Dare to be different. Want to be the change you seek. From the moment you wake up, you have this incredible opportunity not only to ignite change in your own life, but also to affect change in others.

Someone in your life may have you convinced you should be or act a certain way that is different than you naturally would be or act. They may have persuaded you to believe in a specific idea that is not loving to yourself or others. For example, I have always been taught to find a profession that makes me large quantities of money, but I only ever wanted to do something I loved, something that made me proud. I also was raised to cover up my body, but what comes naturally to me is to embrace my nudity and my natural state. So many people are in hiding because they are afraid to lose the approval of others. I don't want to be addicted to the approval of others; I want to follow my heart. I do not want to follow other people's ideas of how they think or believe I should live my life. I am not a follower of people.

The "follower" or "sheep" mentality has been in place since

civilization began. Why do you think trends are so popular? The power of one person's beliefs can change an entire nation. Don't be a follower, be the leader in your own life. Dare to be different, break the mold, and you won't regret it!

INTRODUCING HAPPY WEIGHT

One Third of the American population is classified as obese.[1] But we are individuals, not statistics. While experts rely heavily on numbers to guide discussions of weight, they seem to forget that people have feelings, and that their weight is most likely driven by their feelings. Weight gain is often a sign of physiological duress caused by a combination of factors, such as work, stress, and life traumas. People can also gain weight because of hormonal imbalances, genetic mutations, or the inability to understand a proper clean-eating style, which comes from the lack of education at school or in the home. Statistics don't reveal enough about individuals and the individual factors that are affecting them.

In this book, you will be addressed as an individual. *Happy Weight* is not about how to lose weight. *Happy Weight* discusses the truth about your body and how it needs to be loved on every level. Loving your body can mean so many different things; from investigating what nourishment your individual body actually needs, down to accepting and loving yourself on an emotional level. The physical and emotional are attached, as everything in the body is connected, nothing is separate, and we are all very different.

Body image, weight loss, health, wellness, and love are linked. None of us can experience happiness with our self until we love the skin we live in. By this I mean, we can't honestly take care of all of our health and wellness needs until we fully understand ourselves and what our needs actually are.

When was the last time you loved every single thing about your life and loved every tiny detail about your body? Can you remember? If you are a woman in need of loving her body in every aspect, then *Happy Weight* is written for you. The mind-body-soul connection is essential for wellbeing in all its forms. *Skinny* is just a buzz word, a physical label that holds no authority in the greater scope of a woman's existence. The purpose of *Happy Weight* is to teach you to open yourself to the world and become free from the prison you have made for yourself and your body.

Through this incredible journey into yourself, your health, and your life, you will learn about vulnerability, confidence, nutrition, body love, and how to find that which makes you happy.

You will learn about achieving your happy weight by saying NO to using scales, pant sizes, and the Body Mass Index (BMI) as tools to judge your worth or dictate how your day will begin. This book will help you to uncover the you that is so desperately seeking to be released; to not be afraid of the world; to not be afraid of change; to accept yourself for exactly who you are; to feel worthy of love and to truly love yourself; to understand your relationship with food.

We, as women, struggle so much with the ideas of perfection and the way things are "supposed" to be. That 'so and so' said it was one way so it must be!

I hope that you learn to decide for yourself what care you need. Even some health care providers don't always have the answers you need. I am not asking you to abandon your medications or your doctor's orders. Doing so would be negligent. I am simply encouraging you to do your homework: investigate your body as a whole, and realize that your doctor might not have all the answers. My hope in writing *Happy Weight* is that it can foster a revolution of women desperately working to change the negative ways they see themselves.

Happy Weight is an idea that one size will never fit all. Break out and do something extraordinary: Go against what you believe to be true in the sense of the illusion of everyday life, without proof, and find what really works for you. For example, try cutting out that food that doctors say gives you more calcium (dairy), but you know it gives you a stomachache.

Reconnect with yourself, practice mindfulness, and use self-knowledge to create the ultimate environment you need for sustainable health. Understand and digest that what you thought you knew about nutrition until now is likely false, and that the human body and mind are adaptable and capable of change at any given moment. You can encourage the release of body imprisonment with self-love and mantras, by reconnecting with nature and truly nurturing yourself above all else.

Happy Weight is not a diet. It is an idea that we, as individuals, are the ones that hold the key to our own health. We are the only ones who own our bodies and can tell their real story.

CHAPTER 1
Happy Weight

To love yourself is to be released from the judgment of others.

My name is Daniele Nicole Della Valle and I am a thirty-two-year-old woman living in the Pacific Northwest. I also happen to be a nutritional therapy practitioner certified by the Nutritional Therapy Association. I have worked for several years in clinical and private settings helping women address the full spectrum of health issues, from autoimmune disease to reproductive dysfunction. I use food based protocols, life style mindfulness, and sometimes whole food supplementation to help them achieve their health and wellness goals. I have a special technique I designed myself, whose tenets include creating a safe space and not judging people. It works quite well. When I stopped forcing people to do things, I was surprised how much they could accomplish because they were doing it for themselves.

Most of the women I have counseled in nutrition first come with immediate issues, but are ultimately concerned about their weight. That is what most of us, unfortunately, think about above all else: Our appearance, and not our health. That is most likely what drew you to purchase this book, right? A bunch of powerful, painted, naked ladies on the cover with a title like *Happy Weight*? The title is not meant to be misleading, but this is not a book about weight loss. This book is more than weight loss, and more than health. This book is THE anti-diet manifesto created to help you find the gateway to your body's happy place. In other words, I am going to help you to STOP DIETING, so you can learn to love your body and learn about your health in the process. I am not just writing this book for you, I am also writing it for myself. I've struggled with my body image for as long as I can remember. Yes, I am a nutritionist with body image issues, go figure. Hi, I'm Daniele, and I have hated my body for a long time.

I'm sure it started around the time I was in elementary school. My first week in fifth grade, a classmate made some bullshit comment asking if I was poor because she had seen me wear the same sweater twice in one week. I still remember what that white cable knit sweater with the blue V-neck collar looked like. It was my favorite sweater. My mother gave it to me, why wouldn't I wear it more than once? I'm not sure that after all these years I would have remembered that sweater if it weren't for that negative memory that attached to it. The sad part is that I had just moved, I didn't know anyone, and this was my first memory of the new town we lived in at the time. Unfortunately, kids just regurgitate hateful language taught by their parents, they don't even know it's cruel. They are completely unaware that you were just scarred for life and they are the one to blame.

The next time I remember feeling personal judgment was when I was eleven. I wanted to wear my first training bra. My grandmother said, "What, with those little mosquito bites?" She laughed, thinking she was being cute. I, on the other hand, was insanely embarrassed as I watched my brothers join and laugh with her. Because of that direct body shaming comment, I spent the next ten years wishing and hoping for a larger bust that never came. The women in my family would joke, back handedly hinting that I was lucky that I wasn't cursed with the "McNulty rack, and that I should be grateful that I was "flat chested". All I really wanted was what all people want, validation, and to feel a sense of belonging. At this point I did not.

These are only a couple of stories, but I can still feel all of the embarrassment I have experienced in my life deep inside my heart. I have been called fat, too skinny, healthy and unhealthy. Every person I have ever known intimately brings my skin up in regular conversations, as if I have no idea that I struggle with it. Thank you captain obvious, I get it, I have bad skin.

I have had perfect strangers tell me that they don't like my hair color, or what I was wearing. I have had random guys put their hand up my skirt because they thought that my wearing a skirt was some sort of invitation. I have had women judge me and, best friends say horrible things about me. I've watched women blatantly lie to me to make me feel less than, only to make themselves feel better.

However, I don't write this book to be a victim of my past, to blame these moments for the pain in my life. This is my story, an anecdote to tell you, some context to show you that I know what that pain feels like. I have cried thousands of tears at the words and actions of others. This book is for both of us, for you and me. This book is for us to leave the past behind and welcome a new beginning, one without the opinions of others. One without the hate or discontent we feel toward a situation. This book is about love and happiness. This book is about finding a place inside of both of us where we can celebrate exactly who we are and love the body we live in. This book is about finding our Happy Weight.

Happy Weight is a state of being, the consciousness of a world without living as a prisoner to our own bodies. It is a pathway of living as our true self and not being categorized as a thing that has to fit into an inhuman mold. As women, we fight almost from birth to live without flaws. We live in a culture where weight is forced on us as the gauge of health and wellbeing. We live in a world that makes us hate ourselves.

Every day some women wake up, and before the day has even begun, the first idea they have about themselves is a negative one. What kind of sick world do we live in that perpetuates and promotes women living in a constant state of self-hatred?

Unfortunately, it is our world, our culture, and our society that makes us feel this way. It's everywhere: billboards, TV, radio, social media, friends, family, significant others . . . It feels as though we cannot escape this life of being overly concerned with our physical appearance. We are obsessed with our weight.

We let the scale dictate our happiness and self-worth. We would do anything to change this dynamic, right? Not really. Most of us think we are fat, we think diets are the answer, and we think being super thin is healthy and the key to our ultimate happiness.

The reality of this nightmare is that our culture, which calls for bigger, faster, stronger, now, is killing us. Instant gratification is costing us our health and our satisfaction with our lives.

We need to learn to embrace the following information:

- The physical and emotional go hand in hand.
- Self-hatred is unhealthy.
- Yo-yo diets and crash diets are unhealthy.
- Being an unrealistic size for our individual body type is unhealthy.

Ask yourself this: What is your health worth without your happiness? Don't you want to love every second of your life? To shed the pain you feel because of someone else's idea of beauty? To wake up every day feeling powerful, beautiful, healthy, strong, and capable of taking on the world? It is possible that you do, but you still base your worth and health on your appearance. If so, why? Why do you buy gimmicks that promise you these things, instead of going on a journey to find yourself?

The answer is fear: Fear of change, fear of indifference, fear of judgment, fear of not knowing where to start or if we are doing it correctly.

As women, we are often our own worst enemies. We make countless excuses as to why we can't do something. We make these stories up in our heads about the worst-case scenarios with the worst possible outcomes. This negativity becomes an endless loop that engulfs us. It becomes who we are. We sabotage our goals by not making it to the gym or yoga class. We say to ourselves, "It's just one meal, I can handle it." That one meal turns into an entire week of binging. After the week is over we hate ourselves for our decisions.

We become beings stuck on a ride of perpetual self-loathing, where the endless life of hating ourselves feels like the only option.

There was a time in our history where a natural curve to a woman was revered. We ate from our gardens instead of supermarkets, and we used ancestral remedies instead of drugs to cure disease. Women were seen as the givers of life, healers, and the peacemakers. The term *goddess* was a part of the language we used to describe women. Women held positions of power. Our early ancestors made idols and statues of the female form. There have been many great empresses, queens, and high priestesses throughout history. But somehow, we ceased to recognize their status. Somehow, we forgot how powerful we are, how capable we can be of fulfilling our deepest wants and desires.

Today we base much of our worth and power on our appearance and size. Our culture is saturated with the idea that women need to look a certain way to be beautiful. We have an unwavering belief that we need to be a specific size to be worthy. We feel the need to diet until we look emaciated in order to be considered healthy, sexy, beautiful, and respected. We deprive our bodies of nutrients through our addiction to quick fixes, such as weight-loss drugs, with little to no thought of how these diets could destroy our bodies. We grossly obliterate the natural version of ourselves to fit our culture's unrealistic expectations about women's bodies. Some women engage in crash dieting, so much so that they destroy their metabolism and thyroid glands in the process. Some women never recover from the effects of those diets. I know women who have gone so far as to lose their lives because of unhealthy dieting.

Why does what our society thinks our bodies are supposed to look like have so much power over us?

Think about this: have you ever seen a group of women line up who are all the same weight, but are all different heights, shapes, and sizes? How do we not see that we are all so different?

How do we not see that ONE SIZE DOES NOT FIT ALL!

Our standards of health and beauty in America are truly disgusting. They are incredibly unrealistic, based on bad science.

The details of where it went wrong is something we will discuss later, but the real question for now is, why? Why did we allow society to make us feel less than? Who is the person that decided we weren't pretty enough, skinny enough, smart enough, brave enough, capable enough to make decisions regarding our own health?

You Always Have A Choice

In all of my years of study, I have come across one primary answer. I have heard leaders speak on the subject, psychologists write about it, yogis preach about it. It is US that are ultimately the criminal, judge, and jury of our physical and emotional fate. It is our emotional state of being that dictates the person we see our self as. It is our choice what foods we decide to eat. As adults, we are primarily responsible for our own happiness, for our state of mind, our health, and our wellbeing.

Processing traumatic emotion is the one occasion in which blame is allowed. It is hard to be calm and introspective if we are still reliving a trauma. The rest of the time, it's on us . . . we are the creators of our reality. No one else. We are responsible for all the decisions we have made and will make. We make the choice to not be happy the way we are. We make the choice to not take care of our bodies.

Ownership is the only way we can accept our reality and learn to understand why we are here. We are here to take ownership.

Ownership And Judgment

This book is not here to blame us for our misgivings or our journey in life. It is not to discount any negative direct or indirect experience we have had regarding our body or sense of self-worth. This book is here to encourage us to take ownership over our life and take control of what is rightfully ours: our choices. Every person has the right to choose her own path, no matter the obstacles. It is time to own our choices and take control of our life. From here on out we will decide how to write our own story. Let's get started.

If we didn't know this before, know now that there is a big difference between making a judgment and observing a medical fact. For instance, telling someone they are fat is making a judgment. Being morbidly obese, however, is a fact that a doctor might share with a patient. These two are not the same. Judging someone versus warning her of a health risk—when it is our job to do so—are two completely different scenarios.

Perception is a game I always play with people, and being the devil's advocate is the role I love most often. To change one's perspective from one side to no side is like a checkmate for me. Take our parents for instance, and their parents before them. They loved to call people fat, chubby, chunky, some sort of farm animal reference, butterball, thunder thighs, or "healthy looking." All of these terms and comments are formed in a singular perspective that is learned and unguarded. They taught each other that these terms were correct and didn't care if they were harmful because they thought that they were somehow "doing you a favor" when they used them.

How many women do we know that have a traumatizing

story or experience that they can pull out immediately when asked "What made you hate yourself or think that you were fat?" So many millions of women have been affected for the rest of their lives by one single interaction or conversation! When I've asked the women I counsel this question, typically they tell me a story about someone they had a deep bond with shaming them. Sometimes it was the words of a complete stranger that damaged their self-esteem. I don't care about the "sticks and stones" child's riddle. Words hurt. They leave scars.

BEAUTY CANNOT BE PUT IN A BOX

The proverb "Beauty is in the eye of the beholder" tells us that beauty cannot be judged objectively, for what one person finds beautiful or admirable may not appeal to another. There is no one right answer of how we should or shouldn't look. This is fact. Women in China bleach their skin because in China, a lighter complexion is a sign of beauty; while some women in the United States spend thousands of dollars a year on tanning and darkening their skin. Every person's idea of beauty is different.

Who makes the rules about our bodies anyway? Is it our parents, their parents, and the people that came before them? Is it our teachers, bosses, spouses, or friends?

The truth is that not a single person on this planet has the actual authority to make a statement against who we are, what we look like, or who we want to be. They can't control how we want to be or how we process our thoughts about our lives and ourselves.

Every single person on this earth is faking it. Our ancestors were basing their reasoning on those that came before them, who were quintessentially also faking it, and often got things wrong. Critical people don't get to decide what works for our bodies or us. They only need to worry about themselves, while we worry about ourselves.

In my own experience, the people I once thought to be the

bearers of all truth showed me that no one is perfect. I have had family members, friends, and coworkers pretend at perfection, while living lives that do not conform to their beliefs. I have heard a friend say they wouldn't be caught dead doing something, and then caught them doing that very thing not a moment later. Hypocrisy is everywhere; it is one strong gauge of imperfection.

Remember, those we believe to hold the power to define us carry their own negative definitions of self. Our friends and family are just as screwed up as we are! NO ONE IS PERFECT! NO ONE HAS IT ALL FIGURED OUT!

Others project onto us the misguided, vicious, perpetual cycle of self-hatred and negativity and sometimes we believe it. This is so horribly sad. Why can't people just communicate how they really feel? Why do we have to bully each other?

If we begin to understand the fallacy of the human condition, we can begin to understand the idea of happy weight. Although finding our happy weight may sound profound and complicated, it is actually the opposite. Finding our happy weight is about power, liberation, and freedom.

Finding your happy weight is about loving yourself unconditionally, validating your deepest emotions, setting boundaries, gaining confidence, being vulnerable, and understanding how to be of healthy mind, body, and soul. It is the ultimate state of being to remind you to take care of the one and only body you have in this life. This is a testament to your body and life. You have the power to make it what you want, without fear.

You're following me, right? Happy weight is achieved when you are deeply connected to your health and happiness without question, without harm, and without toxicity.

Change Is Not As Scary As You Think

It is likely that the thought of not being skinny enough has crossed your mind. This act of judgment and self-hatred is regularly justified by the pressures of society to be more. You become overwhelmingly concerned that your worth is not enough. The thought is, *If I were skinnier, my life would be better. I would, in turn, be happier. I would find that magical love of life. I would finally find the greatest happiness to ever exist.*

Upon occasion, I become delusional and think, *I will become prettier, better, and happier if I were skinnier.* Quickly, I wake up and realize that's not reality, that's not how this works. Do I actually think that all skinny people have the answer to life? That when the fat melts away I could become a super being that is shielded from negativity? Not so much. Skinny people have their problems too.

Don't get me wrong. This book isn't about skinny shaming. Or fat shaming, for that matter. I am only making a statement that being skinny may not necessarily mean healthy. This is a profound awakening that size doesn't matter. Your health is your health, be it mental or physical.

You are beautiful no matter what you look like. The prettier, the better, the happier you, already exists, you just have to believe in it- and then own it.

Why is it that life doesn't just magically get better when we lose weight? Because this idea that we aren't thin enough, good enough, attractive enough, happy enough, all stems from something deeper. The deep-seated emotional need to be something that we think we aren't came from something outside of us. It was direct or indirect, either way, we feel unworthy in some way, shape, or form. Somewhere, somehow, we learned not to like the way we look or feel about ourselves.

Has this happened to you? Somehow, you began to believe that your body image was more important than your health. Maybe you saw the recognition another person got and thought, *I want to be treated like that.* Or you had a medical professional tell you that you are in the incorrect weight category, saying, "You need to lose weight." It could be someone in your life that shames you with negative language and bullies you into thinking you will never be good enough. There are so many possibilities.

You may have forgotten that most people are rude and judgmental, and that the idea of "skinny" or "pretty" is created by unrealistic ideals and false promises by other, self-hating individuals. I know that is a mouthful, but whoever is delivering you a plate of self-hatred is not your friend. If they are your friend, family, co-worker, or spouse, they are using projective language.

Projective Language Reveals Insecurity

Projective language comes from a place of personal discourse. "Psychological projection is a theory in psychology in which humans defend themselves against their own unconscious impulses or qualities (both positive and negative) by denying their existence in themselves while attributing them to others."[1]

An example of projection is a mother that raises her daughter with comments like, "You're too fat to wear that," or "Are you going to eat that, my little piggy?" These comments come from a deep place of personal insecurity. These comments are generated from the mother's personal self-hatred and she expresses herself by projecting her own insecurities onto her daughter. Sometimes it isn't a mother or father; sometimes it's someone we thought was a friend.

The person using the language has their own damage they are dealing with. Because this person only knows how to express him or herself through negative language, they will, unfortunately, never heal. They will not heal until they decide to take an introspective approach to life. Only an introspective person has the power to change their mental state. Don't be angry with that person; instead focus on yourself. You can't fix their crazy. That's their job.

The False State Of American Measurement

Where do we get our standards of weight and size from, anyway? We thought scales, measurements, and BMIs were the best measurements we had. These may have been initially created for scientific study, but we do not need to be treated like lab rats. Remember that the physical and emotional go hand in hand. As we came to rely more and more on these measurements, we became emotionally dependent on them to dictate our ultimate happiness. We became a number instead of a person. We began relying on numerical measurements and not personal accomplishments. We began rewarding with food and using words like "treats" and "cheats," making food pleasure seem like some sort of perverse act. Doctors, nutritionists, and personal trainers have a hard time letting go of numerical scales because they truly believe it measures success.

The success of what? Losing and gaining the same weight over and over for the rest of our lives because we have never learned how to truly measure our success. I know almost any doctor, nutritionist, or personal trainer reading this will disagree and say, "Well, according to this study . . . blah blah blah." I have little to no faith in the standard teachings of the American Medical Association. So, if a doctor thinks that weight loss is the only hope, it might be time for them to go to a Functional Medicine or Integrative Health school and take some psychology classes on disordered eating. Health is so much bigger than a black and white approach to fat vs. thin. There is a huge gray area. The human body is made up of so much more than fat tissue, and shaming people into crash dieting will only cause more damage in the long term. Shaming tactics make us feel stuck, and lost, and leave most of us worse off than when we started.

Maybe we think it is normal to be treated differently because of our size? Maybe at some point, someone made us feel less than worthy. Did we think that whoever made us feel less than worthy had the authority to do so? Why?

And why do we so desperately want to be any different than we are? Why are we more concerned about our size and looks, than our health? Why is vanity our driving factor, and not how we feel about ourselves emotionally, as whole people? Being a person is not an abstract idea. Why isn't our primary concern our health and wellbeing?

Why aren't we more concerned with healing our digestion, getting off our medications, sleeping better, or having more energy? Some of us think about having surgery on our hips and knees, when we could easily avoid surgery by healing our bodies.

HEAL WITHIN

What I am trying to say is that how we feel physiologically needs to be the ultimate and primary focus when thinking about our bodies. Not our media-driven, societally approved, negative idea of beauty. Using makeup, plastic surgery, and body-modifying clothing will not hide what is really happening on the inside. Last time I checked, lip injections don't fix emotional trauma.

Do we really want to be just like that one girl on Instagram, that Fitspo queen? Do we think that because she looks a certain way that her life is better? I get that role models are important, but why does the inspiration have to come from someone that looks nothing like us? Unless it is solely for workout routines, nutrition, or lifestyle advice, why are we following them?

Do our role models actually know what they are doing? What makes them credentialed? Is it because they are fit and surviving on 500 calories a day?

That can't be right. If anything, some of these "health coaches" are trained in destroying our health. Do they understand how the endocrine system actually works? They may know nothing about the long-term damage their advice does to the thyroid gland, which is the primary driver of metabolism. Or to our adrenal glands, that control our stress response. If we become so fatigued we will end up right back where we started or much worse.

A personal trainer that uses packaged products as "nutrition" recommendations is someone I want nothing to do with. Unless trainers are preaching that we eat real food, I want no part in their lessons.

Consider what makes you so prone to listening to all of this nonsense. Is your poor body image helping you make poor life decisions?

Do You Like Being Unhappy?

When did you begin to believe that being objectified was better than being what you really are? Can you remember the first time you felt like you weren't "enough?" Who made you feel that way? When did it happen? How did you respond? Do you even remember how it happened? At what point did you become consumed by the idea that being thin would magically make your life better?

If we think the fat on our bodies is repulsive, then we become repulsive to ourselves. We create a cycle of self-hatred and unhappiness. As this continues, desperation sets in and we reach the point where we will do anything to be skinny, believing this is the key to finally being happy with the way we look and feel. We actually start to believe that being skinny will make us happy. We let the scale dictate our happiness and we start to base our worth on a number.

The Insanity

Is that why we are on that liquid shake diet that makes us starve, or that cayenne cleanse that makes our brain feel like it's melting? Is that why we are on that pregnancy hormone diet where we eat 500 calories a day only to gain all our fat tissue back instantly?

How sustainable is that? Were we able to maintain it? How many times have we lost and gained the same weight? When we were at our lowest weight, were we actually happy? Do we believe that being thin makes us happy?

My heart breaks. The truth is, you are already the most amazing person you know. And if you aren't sure that's true, you just haven't met the true you yet.

WHEN DID WE BECOME SO DISCONNECTED?

Why did we stray so far away from our connection to natural foods? When did we begin to rely so heavily on these chemical imitations of real food? How did we lose the intelligence of listening to our own bodies and knowing when something was wrong? The truth is that we forgot to focus on eating **real** food. One day, food became more of a science project than it did sustenance. We started counting calories and fat instead of nutrients.

I had a client bring me a loaf of bread that had over twenty-five ingredients in it and she asked me to help her read the label. I told her that her first mistake was that the front of the package lists calories and fat. The second is that bread should never have more than five ingredients in it, and those five ingredients should be flour, water, yeast, baking soda, and salt. That's it. Unless she was gluten free, and then wheat flour is nowhere to be found. Her third mistake was that nowhere on the package did it say whether or not the food is organic, non-GMO, or minimally processed. The "loaf of bread" was really a loaf of crap. Not because I think so, but because our bodies think so. The organic, non-GMO, gluten-free labels are not a fad; they are a red flag signaling the reality of the world we live in. The reality that we stopped caring about what we put in our bodies because we are so focused on convenience.

In Chapter 3, about nutrition and bioindividuality, I'll get into the how and why, but for now let's explore the shift that desperately needs to take place. The need to clean up how we eat and get back to basics.

Bioindividuality is a word that will appear a lot in this book. It is the idea that every single person is different, and that we all have different approaches to achieving optimal health and wellness. We all have different scopes of understanding, different backgrounds. We all have different genetic makeups. We are all living in different economic, geographic, and physical environments. The result is that no one person on this planet has the exact same biological map. However, the one consistent factor, the common denominator in all of this is the need to eat real, clean, food as medicine, and understand the delicate state of the human microbiome. The Human Genome Project defines the microbiome as "the collective genomes of the microbes (composed of bacteria, bacteriophage, fungi, protozoa and viruses) that live inside and on the human body. We have about ten times as many microbial cells as human cells."[2]

Our microbiome can be altered by the foods we eat. The old saying "you are what you eat," could not be any more real. Eating clean is the best place to start when understanding our effect on our microbiome for the first time. Eating organic, grass-fed, unprocessed foods that are not full of chemicals and additives is the one unchanging variable in human health. We simply forgot how to eat, care about, and pay attention to real, natural foods. The American need for bigger, faster, stronger, and right now has destroyed the culture of slow eating, growing our own food, and nurturing our soul through every aspect of mindfulness.

Mindfulness is one of the most important acts in human existence. Mindfulness is paying attention to any and all of the actions, choices, and movements we make in our lives. As our physical health collectively began to deteriorate, so did our collective mental state of being. Mindfulness has been long forgotten by our culture and we now live in ignorance. We cannot begin to understand how to make changes unless we understand where our ignorance came from.

SHAMING

Unfortunately, the state of emotional health and the systems to support it in our country are declining. How can we begin to process what is ultimately wrong with the physical health of our society if we, as a whole, feel shamed and defeated? How can we begin to rebuild and support each other as a community if we don't believe in ourselves? The American food culture and body shaming go hand in hand. We cannot find our happy weight physically if we do not first begin to heal the wounds of our past.

I recently had a client that came to see me to discuss fat loss. She knew it would not be quick because she wanted, above all, to be healthy. I thought, "Great, a client that has come to terms with her reality." It wasn't until she began to hesitate with making simple changes that I realized she had not fully dealt with the pain of her past, and in particular, the relationship she had with her mother. She was combative and abrasive. She said she was fine, but her face would become flushed any time I suggested a shift or reason why she was not working toward her personal goals. Her deprivation gave her a sense of entitlement. This deprivation came from an all too familiar memory of someone using shaming and abusive language about her body.

Her truth was, how could she expect to make a change in her health or the way she approached her relationship with food if she didn't change the way she viewed herself?

Our food ignorance comes from a history of self-doubt, shaming, guilt, bad habits we were taught, and poor science making us prisoners to toxic products. We resist making food changes because we cannot accept that we are living with a lifetime of shame and a complete lack of vulnerability. True vulnerability is the act of asking for what you want regardless of what others think.

If we do not work through our shame and guilt with vulnerability and gain confidence in the process, we are destined to repeat the past. We will never find completeness if we first do not come to terms with our reality, and work through the pain of the shaming language that was used against, and imprisons us.

We can learn best from living our life with vulnerability and transparency. We can work through the shame by living our truth and making no apologies.

I never push change on my clients. I deliberately never make them feel as though they "have to" or "should" do anything. Health and happiness are a state of mind. Weight is not always the primary factor when it comes to health; fat tissue and the buildup of toxins are. Several recent studies show that some people's buildup of fat tissue can be protective against environmental toxins and oxidative stress.[3] The primary concern here is inflammation and toxin build up, not weight. If we suffer from inflammatory conditions and weight gain, losing the weight may not necessarily correct the issue. The fat itself is not the cause of our disease, the imbalance is. Weight gain is far from the biggest problem in the grand scheme of your health. Inflammation, estrogen dominance, cortisol build up, uric acid build up, and acidic blood are some of the many issues that threaten our health. Some women might actually gain weight as they get healthier, and some may lose weight as a result of their body adapting to a protocol to correct their health. Fat tissue on the body is not the primary identifier of poor health, the existence of an inflammatory disease is. Don't be so quick to compare yourself to or judge another person based on size, they might be healthier than you are.

THE SECRET

The secret to life is: LIVE IT. Be conscious in this life, be mindful, and pay full attention to the world around you. It has nothing to do with how fat or skinny you are. The body you live in is a vehicle to get you through your life, so that you have the chance to experience it. Think of your body as an organic machine house for your consciousness.

We can't float around as consciousness, so this organic machine house helps us see, taste, smell, touch, and experience life. What we look like is not something we can control. Therefore, we can try and contour our bodies as much as we want, but in the end, what we get is what we get. Every single human on this planet is beautifully constructed. We are all so different. So many shapes, sizes, and colors. It is truly amazing. We are incredibly intricate beings. Yet, we have unlearned that our organic machine house needs to be healthy in order for us to continue to experience life.

Have you ever heard "Your body is your temple"? Well, this is truth. Your body is your sanctuary.

This journey through discovering your happy weight will help you understand how to treat your temple. It is about finding yourself and understanding the concept of existing fully. Happy weight isn't just a journey into discovering your true health, it is about finding your voice, being vulnerable, saying NO, and saying YES. The path to finding your happy weight follows these simple themes:

- Establishing confidence and vulnerability

- Nourishing your body's bioindividuality with nutrition

- Stress management

- Losing the guilt

- Breaking up with foods through mindfulness

- The art of saying no

- Creating yourself by finding your tribe

- Detoxifying your home and life

- Ultimately learning how to listen to your beautiful body

This book is a guide to stepping into the amazing woman that you have always been. It is about making her known to you and to the world. Let me be your guide. You may not like me at times, but don't put me down. I promise I will be here every step of the way.

CHAPTER 2
The Journey To Happy Weight

No matter where you are in your journey, you are exactly where you need to be.

Oprah Winfrey

"I am ultimately beautiful, inside and out." This is not something I have always said about myself. As a young person with the many unfortunate interactions I had and remember, I wasn't conditioned to believe so. We are a product of our experiences, good or bad.

In my life, I was always the "new kid." I went to eleven schools before college even though neither parent was in the military. Because of the constant changes, I became an extremely timid and shy child, like a scared dog that needed a lot of reassurance. My parents wanted me to believe that everything was always okay, but in time I realized they were hiding, what they thought was the ugliest part of their life, from me, to protect me. I felt really confused by this.

Now being an adult, as a rule, I rely on being told the truth because deception—even if it is mild and well intentioned—makes me feel out of control. I realized much later in life that truth is subjective. In trying to disguise the imperfections in their lives, people routinely hide their true selves and in doing so, deny themselves of connection with one another.

Had they known at the time that I was capable of understanding our circumstances and would still see them as the amazing people that I love, maybe their efforts would have been less of a feeling of self-loathing and regret. However, vulnerability does not come easy to everyone.

Vulnerability can most often be a person's greatest enemy. When we are incapable of living in our truth, we live in half-truths and lies, and we create new stories so we don't have to live in the life defined by our old ones.

We as adults tend to believe that others cannot handle our truth, or better yet that we cannot truly handle others knowing it. In my eyes my parents and grandparents did their best raising us with every experience possible. They gave us the gift of family.

Growing up, my dad took us on every adventure he could think of, while my mom made sure we were as active as possible with skiing, hiking, rock climbing, and surfing. We spent every summer with my grandparents in southern Oregon making fudge, fishing, camping, and picking blackberries for jam. Those summers gave me the consistency I so desperately craved and I found myself yearning for simpler times. Because we moved so much, I grew up feeling confused and displaced; I had nothing in common with the kids in my schools. It was really hard for me to make more than a few friends in fear that we would be moving shortly thereafter. My one wish would be to go back and fully understand our circumstances. Instead my parents chose to live in half-truths, and I was never given the whole story. I had to piece things together on my own and formulate my own opinion. I never knew we moved for monetary reasons. Selflessly my parents never let us want for anything even if they had no money. I live with guilt thinking about how many times my siblings and I so selfishly asked for more, when we did nothing to help the situation. We were the definition of spoiled children, but I never wanted to be one. It wasn't what I cared about; I wanted to know the truth. Being poor would never have bothered me, I'm not a materialistic person. Had I known, maybe I would have understood more about why my parents were in such a state of disarray for so long. It would have drastically changed how we affected one another's lives. The pain, frustration, confusion, and expectation that still exists amongst my siblings and parents could have been diffused. Honesty and vulnerability go deeper than you think. It is all I needed. It is all we ever need.

"The truth will set you free," a quote to live by. Once we stand in our truth, there are no unanswered questions, we don't live with the guilt or shame of memories we don't understand, we aren't left feeling as though our story doesn't make sense.

I also wasn't raised to know that people are cruel and hateful. I didn't know that people would try to selfishly influence their opinion every chance given. I was so mesmerized by every idea and thought, I would do exactly what people expected of me. The expectation was insurmountable, it was deafening. Before I learned to change, I was a product of my environment. I listened to anything and everything people said. I thought they were being honest, telling the truth, not just forcing their selfish opinion on me. I became a joke to people, they would say, "Daniele will believe anything you tell her, she's so gullible."

I think now, *is it wrong to want people to be honest with me, or themselves?* When I was in my teens and early twenties some of my closest friends began to hide things from me. I think they felt as though the truth would hurt too much. When the truth was eventually revealed, they were the only ones hurt- they were the ones that had to deal with *their* truth. My whole life people have lied to my face, with complete confidence. Friends, family, clients, complete strangers. For what? Fear of their reality. Fear that they will not be seen as an equal. Ego.

Now, instead of growing into an untrustworthy person, I am a more conscientious person. I have tried to become more of a human lie detector. I watch body language, tones, eye contact, I recall past conversations. I am always listening, watching, and waiting. I do this because humans are fallible, as we've discussed. Now I ask the right questions and don't take anyone at face value. Most people aren't just lying to others, they are constantly lying to themselves. Most people refuse to live in their truth.

If people can't live in their truth, sadly they will try and push their insecurities on to you. This causes people to force opinion and try to alter your choices.

To believe everyone or everything is dangerous, it can dictate the choices we make in life, it can influence us to our very core. Hear this: *to believe anyone holds truth or power over who we think we are is to be tricked by the game of life.* Listening to intuition, to our gut, is how we can break free from these opinions. Opinions are not truth; they are driven by the conviction of others. When we learn to see through these opinions, the real truth comes to light about our environment. And the real truth is this: we can change whatever we want, whenever we want about our life, in a very real way.

Growing up in southern California, I knew a lot of women who would do anything to lose weight and would then lie about it. It was not an ideal environment to foster healthy body image. I've also known men that couldn't help but think women were supposed to look a certain way and pushed their ideas on others, leaving emotional scars. It left many scars for me. I distinctly remember being called thunder thighs, mosquito tits, and funny face. I don't blame those people for their actions or their own poor body image. They couldn't help what was passed down to them, or was caused by growing up in our American culture. I distinctly remember weight being a part of most conversations regarding how someone was doing. "Oh hey, how is so and so?" "Oh well, you know, she looks like she gained twenty pounds."

The sad truth, that I regretfully admit, is that I was at the other end of many of these conversations. I, too, was conditioned to base someone's general condition on her weight. I thought it was normal because I watched all of the women around me say it. It wasn't until I understood what it felt like to be simultaneously shamed and the shamer- did I begin to take stock. It is absolutely inhumane and disgusting behavior to judge a person by the way they look; to define a person and who they are because of their size. However, millions of people do it every day, and we allow it. I allowed it.

I allowed people to tell me to put makeup on because they thought I looked better with it. They had no shame in telling me that. I allowed people to tell me I wasn't creative, simply because I didn't fit their mold of creativity. I allowed people to shame me into what I thought was motivation, but was purely body shaming, thus creating a binge cycle that was destroying my health. We all allow it. We give others full permission to dictate how we feel about ourselves.

We are also guilty of judging ourselves when people simply ask, "How are you doing?" Instead of thinking of positive things to say, we focus on the negative. "I feel fat today." "Ugh, I could swear I've gained ten pounds." "I'm having a bad hair day." "My job sucks." "I'm stressed."

Who wants to live in a world where this is how we respond to "How are you today?" Not me.

WAKE-UP CALL

I woke up one day and asked myself: *Is this how I really want to live my life? Do I want to greet people with "Life sucks" every time I see them? Is this all I have to look forward to: constant self-hatred, a negative outlook, and negative establishment in conversation? Negative, negative, negative?* No thanks. I wanted to lead a life of joy, love my body, feel elated when I meet people, and leave them feeling fulfilled. I didn't want my mark in life to be anything but full of love and intention. I didn't want people at my funeral to remember me as someone who just couldn't get it together, and only talked about how fat her ass was, or was stricken with a victim mentality. What I am saying is: don't live a life of regret. Don't wait until you are dying to reflect on a life you could have lived more mindfully and fulfilled.

Norway

I can only remember one time in my life when I felt as though my body was never judged. When I was fifteen, I made the decision to study abroad, and moved to Norway.

Before I committed to this life-altering journey, my outlook was very simple. I believed everything everyone told me was fundamentally true. I lived a life of pure, ignorant bliss. I thought that everyone in the world had the same perspective as the people that surrounded me. I thought that the world was how I saw it, and that I was destined to feel like I didn't belong. I had no idea how wrong I was.

It was like I had been asleep for sixteen years. It wasn't until I felt truly accepted that I realized that life was nothing like I had imagined. I thought that I would be a prisoner of my existence until the end of time. It was by no means an easy year. Challenging a person's idea of life, body image, community, family, education, and independence—these are all jarring and traumatic. The trauma, however, wore off as I gained more experience. The more ideas I was introduced to and the more experiences I had, the more hunger I felt for life, learning, and growing. At the end of my year, not having noticed during my almost-eleven-months' stay, I had gained weight. I had no idea I was gaining weight because no one had said anything about it. Not one person made me feel like I needed to be anything other than myself. My amazingly sweet, loving, and nonjudgmental Norwegian girlfriends never once made a comment regarding my body. They only encouraged me to be my best self. The challenges they gave me were always social and academic. My happiness and intelligence were the only concerns of my bad-ass Viking babes. They encouraged me by no longer speaking English in my presence so I could learn Norwegian. They made me feel comfortable enough to shower with all the other girls after gym class, instead of using the solo period shower. I used the solo shower because, when I first arrived, I was too shy to shower around other people. I was so afraid of letting others see my body, I was ashamed. My Norwegian girls changed me, changed my idea of my body. They made me feel like I belonged, they never made me feel like I wasn't worthy or good enough. I will never forget their kindness, and their support. I gained more weight than I was used to and I loved my body more in that moment naked in the shower, where others could see me, and I didn't care. I was empowered to be, just me. This experience of true sisterhood shaped the way I began to treat other women. Now I try to compliment them always, to make them feel safe and comfortable, because I remember what it was like to feel fear and disgust. Now I feel free and beautiful.

This dream like state was almost squandered. It wasn't until my family came to visit at the end of the year that I realized my body had changed for what my biological family and Californian friends saw as the worst they had ever known me to look. This was the first time in my life I had ever gained weight, and when it was brought to my attention, my perception of my body at the time went completely downhill. I felt ashamed, I felt disgusted, I felt as though I had done something wrong, like I had committed a crime against humanity. I was sixteen years old. I had gained 30 pounds of body fat. I am not going to go into detail of the comments made, because I don't blame my family for what they said. They didn't know better. This was a direct result of the way their parents, friends, and colleagues view the body, and how they truly believe that this shaming language is appropriate. I will only say that they made me feel unworthy. After a year of being apart, our first encounter was uncomfortable and traumatizing. I blame myself for allowing them to make me feel any negativity about my body and not to continue feeling as beautiful as I felt before their arrival. It was that contrast that really opened my eyes and I promised to never be the villain in my own story, and that I would dedicate my life to service and lifting others to the highest esteem.

So, regardless of all the negativities I felt in that last week of my life in Norway, my whole life, as I knew it, began to change. Something was set in motion, something was different, I was different. I was never the same after Norway. My eyes were open to the world; I saw that beauty was truly skin deep. I realized that literally ANYTHING could be achieved if you are determined to accomplish it. My host parents were quite different from my biological parents, not better, just different, they were strict, but followed up on results. They pushed me to my limits, but I was stronger because of it. By the end of my year there I was conversationally fluent in Norwegian and dreaming in this new, foreign language. My mind had been forever expanded. It was really hard to get re-acclimated. I felt as though I didn't belong when I came back to the states. Almost like I had always been an outcast, but I just hadn't been far enough away to see it. I really tried to do the normal things my friends back home did, but it never really clicked for me. My awareness and consciousness came alive for the very first time and I will be forever grateful and indebted to those involved in my life there.

The In-Between

The next few years it was hard to feel as though I had purpose, I felt lost, I felt ultimately concerned with the approval others, mostly the people I dated. I didn't belong. I went to college and I studied abroad again, this time a blissful year in China, which was also an amazingly loving, challenging, and encouraging experience. I worked a million different jobs, all in food service and hospitality. I wasn't interested in the day-to-day grind that most people succumb to; I was hungry for something else. I was on that path for about ten years. When I was twenty-six,

I decided to make a choice that was solely my own, unattached, untethered, no friends in tow, no male prospects in wanting. I was free. For the first time since I had left Norway and China, I felt as though I belonged somewhere, like I had finally come home.

I think I felt at home, because Portland, Oregon is a place where people are fighting for social justice, body positivity, and equality. It was around this time when I had the distinct realization that I was a child of the earth and that I just wanted others to be happy in exactly who they are.

STARTING TO HELP MYSELF AND OTHERS

After a decade or so of trying every eating plan--vegan, low carb, low fat, paleo, eating out, cooking at home, binging, yo-yoing, crash dieting--I realized that this couldn't be the answer. I was hungry for more information. My godmother was a Nutritional Therapy Practitioner (NTP) and thought that it would be a good idea for me to become one as well. I agreed, so I decided to go back to school to become an NTP.

I thought it would take ages to find a job in nutrition, but the universe had other plans. My first job out of school was with a holistic ketogenic weight loss company. The ketogenic diet is defined as "a high-fat, adequate-protein, low-carbohydrate diet that in medicine is used primarily to treat difficult-to-control (refractory) epilepsy in children. The diet forces the body to burn fats rather than carbohydrates."[1] The holistic aspect was how the clinic used whole food supplementation, and was focused on natural approaches. This job was simultaneously the best, and the worst possible place for me. I was quickly thrown into the depths of the psyche of the modern American women trying to lose weight. She is made up of all shapes, sizes, colors, backgrounds, religions, cultures, and health histories. America is a melting pot of vast differences. This experience was life changing.

After almost two years of ten-hour days and counseling almost twenty women in a given day about nutrition and education of body process, I had a crash course in what Malcolm Gladwell's *Outliers* describes as my 10,000 hours to mastery.[2] I don't know if I actually achieved 10,000 hours, but it sure felt like it. After a lifetime of having a poor personal body image, after listening to the intimate insights the women around me expressed, I finally understood the answer. It was the answer to everything. Our SELF-LOVE is controlled by our MENTAL and PHYSICAL WELLBEING.

If we are emotionally and physiologically healthy, then we will find our happy weight. If we harbor any negativity towards others, or ourselves or experience unrest, we will never find our bliss, we will never be satisfied.

NUTRITION TRUTHS

Imagine that everything you knew to be true about nutrition and dieting is false. Imagine that low-fat diets and calorie restrictions are wrong, and that doctors and scientists have made a huge mistake. What would you do?

The likely reaction would be shock, awe, concern, and a feeling that it's too late and that the damage has been done. Perhaps utter disbelief and an inability to move past what you thought to be true. That was how I felt.

Now understand, you have been lied to. Understand that the truth about dieting and nutrition is that there is no one right answer. One size never fits all.

The sad truth of all of this is that the people we thought we could trust, our health care providers, have lost their way. There were many physicians so concerned with promoting new drugs and overmedicating us that they forgot how to be real practitioners. Some practitioners forgot to continue researching, and growing their knowledge. They forgot to protect us. These general practitioners became so stuck in their ways that they made it a priority to make us feel as though they are superior to us. Through doctor visits and our cultural belief that doctors know everything about health, we began to believe that our understanding of our own body is false. But is it?

The Hippocratic Oath that all doctors swear to when receiving their medical degrees states[3]:

> *I swear to fulfill, to the best of my ability and judgment, this covenant:*

> *I will respect the hard-won scientific gains of those physicians in whose steps I walk, and gladly share such knowledge as is mine with those who are to follow.*

> *I will apply, for the benefit of the sick, all measures [that] are required, avoiding those twin traps of overtreatment and therapeutic nihilism.*

> *I will remember that there is art to medicine as well as science, and that warmth, sympathy, and understanding may outweigh the surgeon's knife or the chemist's drug.*

> *I will not be ashamed to say "I know not," nor will I fail to call in my colleagues when the skills of another are needed for a patient's recovery.*

> *I will respect the privacy of my patients, for their problems are not disclosed to me that the world may know. Most especially must I tread with care in matters of life and death. If it is given me to save a life, all thanks. But it may also be within my power to take a life; this awesome responsibility must be faced with great humbleness and awareness of my own frailty. Above all, I must not play at God.*

> *I will remember that I do not treat a fever chart, a cancerous growth, but a sick human being, whose illness may affect the person's family and economic stability. My responsibility includes these related problems, if I am to care adequately for the sick.*

> *I will prevent disease whenever I can, for prevention is preferable to cure.*

> *I will remember that I remain a member of society, with*

special obligations to all my fellow human beings, those sound of mind and body as well as the infirm.

If I do not violate this oath, may I enjoy life and art, respected while I live and remembered with affection thereafter. May I always act so as to preserve the finest traditions of my calling and may I long experience the joy of healing those who seek my help.

I don't know about you, but this is not what I experienced at the doctor's office growing up. Only a handful of physicians I have seen have ever given me sympathy, understanding, compassion, or control. The American Medical Association has some fairly awful people representing them.

Not all are horrible. There are some amazing physicians on the front lines of change, the ones continuing to grow, and being the change they seek. These physicians guide us toward a more natural approach, they don't push surgery or pills, and they truly want us to succeed. We aren't a dollar sign to them.

On the flip side, the amount of over medicating that is happening in our country, and the faulty diagnoses, are devastating. When I was ten years old, I was put on a prescription of Tagamet for gastritis. What followed were years of pain due to a faulty diagnosis. Again and again I would be victim to overly prescribed drugs and was not once given a nutrition protocol. When I was seventeen, I was put on six sets of antibiotics, back to back, for a simple bronchial infection. This destroyed my gut health even more than it already had been. The true cause of all of my issues was that I was born with food sensitivities, poor gastric juice production, and an improperly populated gut bacteria. The easy fix would have been to remove a few foods, take zinc, and probiotics. Instead, I spent my life sick after almost every meal and was told it was all in my head. Not a single person advocated for me. And why? Because my physicians stopped doing their own investigations and started to be run by big pharmaceutical interests. They educated parents that everything was "fine" or "normal." The biggest health devastation in modern human history is the American medical agenda over the last seventy years.

I do not, however, place the blame on those who didn't know better, those who were ignorant to the reality that was possible. As I said before, those who came before them conditioned my doctors, my parents, and my teachers.

Because scientific research hasn't discovered our limitless potential, our finite reality is what we have been programmed to believe in. "Because science says so" is not an answer. Science changes every day. Our understanding of the human body today is completely different from what it was seventy years ago, so why do we still believe in the same dietary restrictions laid out in the 1950s and 1960s? Our food pyramid is updated frequently, yet we are still being brainwashed by an idea that is unreasonably outdated. Have you even thought to challenge some of the ideas you hear from "health experts"? Probably not. The thought is that "oh, so and so said this, so it must be true." That is a very dangerous way to live. We are giving perfect strangers full permission over the health and wellbeing of OUR bodies...

When Did We Lose Control?

What happened to us that we felt the need to plague ourselves with the idea that we are not good enough? When did the doctor become the only authority on health, the end all be all? When did nutritionists, weight loss specialists, or diet experts, learn more about our bodies than we know? Who told us that we needed to be on a diet in the first place? Since when did we become lifetime members at a weight loss company? What happened to us? When did we lose so much control over our own health and wellness? How is it that we have come so far in modern history, yet we let society control our every move?

These are all great questions that everyone should be asking more often. In my opinion we stopped learning how to sustainably eat and take care of ourselves. We have been thrown into this horrible, constant yo-yo dieting cycle of weight gain and weight loss. We will reach our weight loss goal, but not know how to maintain it. These programs don't teach sustainability, because they are motivated by profits, and we gain the weight back only to want to lose the same weight again.

It's not our fault and we shouldn't feel guilty about any of this. It is human nature to be trusting of those we believe to be in our corner. We stand up for those who present themselves to be kind and helpful. Like that doctor we have been seeing for twenty years or that weight loss center that always calls us by our first name. We trust, and we give our lives to people that we think have our best interests at heart. The reality is that we are puppets in a larger game. The game is about keeping us in the dark, keeping us from the truth about our health, and how we can be the masters of our own lives.

The weight loss and supplement industry is a billion-dollar industry, so is the cancer industry. The pharmaceutical companies want us to be sick and take their drugs, that is how they profit. Humans have become customers of body commodity. The sicker we are, the wealthier they become.

Think about it. The next time your doctor suggests you take something, find out what it does in the body. Why are you taking it? Was your doctor a part of the drug trial? Did a pharmaceutical sales representative, without a medical background, come in to wine and dine your doctor until they bought a drug they really know nothing about?

Gerald Roliz, author of *The Pharmaceutical Myth*, is a former pharmaceutical company representative turned certified nutrition consultant, or CNC. He uncovers the truth about drug companies and the drugs themselves.

His story is quite fascinating; in his book, he goes deep into how drug reps get doctors to buy more pharmaceuticals. It is like a game the doctors play to get "taken care of" so to speak, and they give the rep whatever he/she wants. Gerald realized quickly that there must be more to life and to medical science.

He discovered the art of using food as medicine and went back to school to become a CNC. His life transformed as he counseled people on the magic of food as medicine. It is a wonderfully thought out beacon of light that blasts Big Pharma out into the open. He decodes the lies of the industry, how much of a "good ol' boys" club it is, and how easily doctors can choose dollar signs over people's health and quality of life.

According to 2013 statistical research done by the Centers for Disease Control, over 50 percent of Americans are currently taking prescription drugs. America is by far the most over medicated country in the world.[4]

In 2015, The Daily Beast released an article stating that Big Pharma is "America's New Mafia."[5]

So what happened to us? How did we lose our way?

THE POINT

What does any of this have to do with the journey to your happy weight? I believe in purpose and I insist on living my life with purpose. I have found this string of patterns through my life that continue to challenge my core beliefs. There are few pieces of advice I have truly taken to heart in my lifetime, but one of them is to always listen. Listen to your heart, listen to your gut, listen to what those around you are saying, and make your interpretation based on how you feel.

THE WHISPERS OF YOUR ANCESTORS

Ancestral health is at the pinnacle of my nutrition philosophy. When clients first come to me for nutrition therapy, they are often only aware that food is sold in grocery stores, restaurants, and fast food establishments. The awareness of where food really comes from has been lost. No one is taught how their body works, what it does, what foods can heal it, and why. There is no shame in this. I get a lot of red, flustered faces, crossed arms, and looks of general anxiety, confusion, and discomfort when I say this to people. This is all normal. I am completely challenging what my clients think they know about food. Change is always uncomfortable.

Before Americans started buying food in boxes and cans, we grew our own. We milked goats, cows, and sheep. We raised chickens for eggs, and slaughtered our own pigs for bacon. We canned and pickled foods. We made broth from bones and used the animal, nose to tail. Life was different. In modern times, our bodies still need the benefits of these practices. Getting back to basics is the answer. Before the 1920s, heart disease was virtually non-existent, much like most diseases today and the excess of pharmaceutical drugs and doctor visits were significantly less than today.[6] There were socioeconomic reasons behind this, and modern medicine and the sciences have evolved to help in immediate situations, but people are now sicker than they ever have been. We currently have the highest rate of heart disease and cancer in comparison to our nation's past.[7] In the book *Nutrition and Physical Degeneration* written by Weston A. Price, it is described that denatured foods like processed grains and sugar are the downfall of human kind.[8] Our ancestors nourished their bodies with bone broths, organ meats, and fermented foods, instead of antibiotics. They stayed fit and healthy by incorporating daily movement, strong community, nutrient-dense vegetables, and sustainably raised meats into their lives. Heart disease, Alzheimer's disease, and cancer were virtually non-existent before the 1900s, because of the art of healing with whole foods.[9] It wasn't the norm for people to have heart attacks at a young age or to suffer from high cholesterol. Doctors didn't need to tell people to lose weight because obesity was such a small problem. Diabetes was also virtually nonexistent. According to recent studies, obesity rates have increased by 214 percent since the 1950s![10] SHOCKING!

The sad truth is that we aren't necessarily eating more. We have just been given poor choices and no education to choose foods that nourish and heal the body. Remember how I mentioned that we love to make communities? Well that's how culture works. One process is set in motion, and then society will eventually adjust and follow. We have followed a set of bad ideas and poorly informed ways of living. All of the processed foods and chemicals we ingest on a daily basis have altered our body's natural state and have destroyed our natural defenses. We are in a constant inflammatory state, increasing our rate of disease. The simplicity of removing processed and inflammatory foods while repopulating a healthy gut can actually reverse disease. Go figure!

The Hippocratic oath was established because the ideas that Hippocrates blessed us with were the reality of the human condition. He stated that we should "Let food be thy medicine, and medicine thy food."[11] Humans can be healed with food. It may seem like bizarre, hippie nonsense, but this our reality. Remember our organic machine house. Organic machines need organic materials to survive. The Franken-crap we are eating is not only killing us, but is also making us hate ourselves in the process.

We have become a nation obsessed with doctor visits and medication, weight loss and diets. We have become obsessed with the idea that a magic pill or program will make us whole again. We make believe that the years of stress, heartache, trauma, and a poor diet will all be erased if we just take that supplement that Dr. Oz recommended, or try that crazy, sugar-filled Master Cleanse diet for thirty days. We actually believe that all of the negativity will just be wiped clean with one, tiny pill. This is the poison we have been fed by our doctors, television, junk food producers, and weight loss companies.

All of this leads us to where we find ourselves today. We're stuck in a vicious cycle of losing, gaining, losing, and gaining. We never feel completely satisfied. Every year, we begin with a fresh start, and for a bit we feel great on our new plan or fad diet. We exercise and drink more water. But somewhere along the line, we stop abruptly. The idea of maintaining the routine becomes too difficult. Maybe we can't continue, emotionally, with the restrictions and so we self-sabotage. The desire to live a normal life gets in the way. For some of us there is an event, a birthday party, a weekend away, or a stressful meeting that breaks our commitment. For others, the new routine loses its luster or seems too restrictive. Either way, we begin to forget. We forget to take care of our body and decide to eat whatever we want. Is it because we have no control, our emotions take over, and then we can't commit? Is it because we have simply given up, or would rather eat our way to a slow and uncomfortable death? Who knows why we give up, or decide to make a million excuses? Everyone is different. Why are we on the diet in the first place? We began with good intentions, so what caused the inspiration to fizzle out?

I ask every single one of my clients during their first visit what diets they have tried in the past. They usually name off the same long list of mainstream fad diets that I have heard before. I pose a second question: "How did they work out for you?" The client then proceeds to tell me that they didn't work and they gained all their fat tissue back. For some, the weight gain was almost immediate. The reasons are sometimes the same, sometimes different. Why aren't any of these diets sustainable? Why is it that these plans don't work, and why are they coming to see me? What answer do I have that they don't?

TRUTH!

You want to know the answer . . . Truth bomb! DIETS DON'T WORK. They don't work because they don't get to the root of why a person gains fat tissue in the first place. They don't get to the root of their body image issues or insecurities, they especially don't deal with eating disorders- they typically create them. This is why my method is easier for people, because I am not forcing anyone to do anything, and I don't put people on diets. I focus on sustainability, not return customers. Happy weight isn't about losing weight; it's about finding a sustainably healthy and happy lifestyle that works for YOU.

The American idea of weight loss is completely wrong. Obesity isn't the issue; it is the behavior and the emotion attached to that behavior. It's also a laundry list of contributing factors such as genetic mutation and expression, gut microbiota, emotional, environmental and oxidative stress, emotional instability, lack of confidence, fear, and sleep disorders caused by all of the above.

The list goes on and on. Do you want to know what your doctor, dietician, and weight loss expert have never told you about? BIOINDIVIDUALITY. You may not be familiar with this word, but the definition in a nutshell is that ONE SIZE NEVER FITS ALL.

Doing a crash diet will never help an emotional eater, and food restrictions will never be sustainable for a binge eater. It is not enough to use tiny containers to educate people on "real portions." The standard portion size might not even be right for our particular body type. There are bigger issues here that no one wants to talk about when putting us on or introducing us to a diet, or discussing our health. These unrealistic programs don't work long term because they aren't there for us in weak or stressful moments, and they don't create change or reset habits that are comfortable. They don't educate us on bigger issues like gallbladder disease, or adrenal fatigue, leaky gut, or inflammation.

The human chorionic gonadotropin (HCG) diet, restricts women to 500 calories a day.[12] Imagine what that does to the body long term. Who actually believes that such restrictions will magically reset their metabolism? How can the body go back to eating 1,500 calories a day after that diet and not gain weight? Don't get me wrong, I'm not blaming anyone has tried this diet. We didn't know better, and trusted the "experts" when they said it would work. But are they really experts? None of these magic diets are sustainable. So, what is the right answer? What is going to help us get healthy and feel good? What is going to get us to stop believing that this time it will be different? The answer is simple. We have to get to know our self from the inside out. Eating a sustainable and healthy diet is 90 percent psychology and 10 percent actually doing it. Following a plan that is restrictive and makes us feel guilty or self-loathing for straying off it is puritanical nonsense. Nobody has time for that!

KNOW YOUR BODY

Before we can fix our broken patterns, we need to first understand how the body actually works. For instance, most people today think they suffer from heartburn because of too much stomach acid. This couldn't be further from the truth. For a majority of Americans, the burning sensation people experience is due to a lack of proper gastric juices and poor digestion caused by stress, inflammation, food sensitivities, prescription medication, acid blockers, or overconsumption of starchy carbohydrates. The best book to read on this subject is *Why Stomach Acid is Good For You* by Jonathan Wright. Stomach acid is essential, but if not taken care of, it can be the leading contributor to health issues. It sounds simple, right? Most gastroenterologists sadly won't tell their patients that.

The hardest part, once we have realized that we have been lied to and overly influenced for our entire lives, is knowing whom we can trust. When women tell me that Google saved their lives after their doctors told them nothing was wrong, I worry that real change within the establishment is hard to find. This is what plagues me at night.

When I sit in a crowded office meeting, making a presentation about nutrition, while everyone around me is eating Jimmy Johns for lunch, thinking, *Oh, it has lettuce in it, it must be healthy*, I worry. Or that time I went to Claim Jumper with some friends after a paintball game and I was the only one not eating or drinking foods that cause damage to my health.

I'm not saying I am superior to anyone, I'm saying that the sad truth is that this is an epidemic. America today is not what it once was when it comes to health. All of our great grandparents and people that came before us lived to be ninety-plus because society and wellness ran a perfect partnership. We drank broth made from bones to nourish us back to health. Life was about being active, constantly outdoors, and socializing. We ate slow meals together for hours and were a part of our community. Life before the 1950s was different. We may not have had our social issues under control, but we knew better when it came to taking care of ourselves. We didn't take an antibiotic every time we were sick. We actually listened to our bodies and knew how to take care of ourselves.

This is why I wrote this book: to try and help you uncover the truth about your own personal health journey and to help you find your happy weight. The truth about wellness and about how the diet and pharmaceutical industries function needs to be explored. The truth about how you are already perfect in every way needs to be embraced. If you want to make a change, let it be on your terms. Learn how to listen to your body and educate yourself on how to take care of it. Stop being a drone to a system that controls the fate of your health.

Let's all work together to stop being zombies, let's wake up!

CHAPTER 3
Bioindividuality

Happy weight is not a diet; it is an idea that we as individuals are the only ones that hold the key to our health.

When discussing health goals and desires of general wellbeing, weight loss should never be the primary goal. What I mean by that is that we seem to go directly to weight loss and physical image instead of taking time to investigate our bodies and truly understand why we are in our current physical and emotional state.

I have had so many clients over the years that refuse to take ownership and understanding of the process, and want a quick solution to reaching their nutrition, wellness, and health goals. They are always looking for that fast fix. Much like the drugs they are given by allopathic doctors, which unfortunately only mask the issues, instead of getting to the root cause. Regardless of the fact that it took a lifetime of damage to arrive at this point, they still think thirty days of taking a pill twice a day is going to do the trick. The primary focus is always a physical manifestation of what they think healthy and happy looks like. There is no desire to understand their body.

As a society, we have a desperate need to understand what is happening inside of our bodies, hormonally, physiologically, mentally, and emotionally. We have a lot of work to do.

This work involves a lot of investigation: investigation of the self, the body, the mind, and the world. How do we actually work as individuals? What makes our bodies function properly, and how are our needs different from another person's needs? It all comes back to food and dieting. We know how we got here, to our extremely distorted idea of beauty standards in America, but what we don't realize is what dieting has done to our foods. We don't realize that the obsession with weight loss and following bad science has started an epidemic food trend of processed, modified foods that no longer nourish us, they only make us sicker. Like the "low fat" diet trend for example. Dietary saturated fats are essential for the body and brain to function properly, yet we cut fat out and now diabetes and Alzheimer's are at an all-time high. The diet industry has destroyed us.

Let's examine the diet industry for a second. When did we start feeling that we needed to be on a diet anyway? When did the brainwashing begin? Diets don't work, so why do we hold onto the idea that they will for so long. Why are we still obsessed with dieting?

The history of binging and purging dates back about 2,000 years[1] if we want to get really focused on when "dieting" began.[1] For Americans, it got a lot more mainstream in 1840 when Sylvester Graham started to recommend a diet of controlling food and restriction.[2] For the next 160 years, we would fall victim to diet trends, pills, shakes, public body shaming, and brainwashed unrealistic expectations propagandized by our own peers. The noise of "you're too fat," or "you're not skinny enough" or "you're too skinny" is deafening; it follows us everywhere. We don't need to be a genius to recognize that American culture has a serious problem when it comes to judgment of physical appearance. Even our so-called "experts" are against us.

Think back to the last time your diet guru told you to get rid of your scale, or stop using measurements, or used photos of unrealistic body types as a tool to encourage you. The truth is, they want you to fail, they want you to hate yourself, and they want you to continue the cycle so that they will make more money off of your self-hatred.

Body dysmorphic disorder, or BDD, is described as, "a mental disorder in which you can't stop thinking about one or more perceived defects or flaws in your appearance—a flaw that, to others, is either minor or not observable. But you may feel so ashamed and anxious that you may avoid many social situations."[3]

Someone suffering from body dysmorphic disorder may intensely obsess over his or her appearance and body image, repeatedly checking the mirror, grooming or seeking reassurance, sometimes for many hours each day. The perceived flaw and the repetitive behaviors cause significant distress, and impact someone's ability to function in their daily life.

They may seek out numerous cosmetic procedures to try to "fix" the perceived flaw. Afterward, there may be some temporary satisfaction, but often the anxiety returns and they may resume searching for a way to fix the perceived flaw."

BDD can also be linked to obsessive-compulsive behavior. The National Eating Disorder Association states that 42 percent of first to third grade girls want to be thinner, 81 percent of ten-year-old girls are afraid of being fat, and one third of all teen girls experiment with various eating disordered behavior. This behavior can include smoking, vomiting, laxative abuse, fasting, or skipping meals.[1] The sad thing is that we aren't born this way. Those around us teach us at an extremely young age, to hate our bodies. Twenty million women today currently struggle with or have experimented with disordered eating.[4] These numbers are of significant proportion to our population.

The outcome of disordered eating is complete system failure and most often death. Slowly, through the emaciation process, the body begins to disease in so many forms. Tooth decay and staining begins, peptic ulcers develop, the bones start to deteriorate, and the rest of the body follows into a severely diseased state.

"Anorexia nervosa is the highest mortality rate amongst all mental illnesses. Between 5% and 20% of people who develop the disease eventually die from it."[5]

I once had a beloved aunt who was the most dedicated, vibrant, and giving woman I have ever met. She officiated my wedding, and I loved her with every ounce of my being. She died earlier this year. I was there. I watched her take her last breath. I felt responsible for not being able to help her. It took months of tears and several powerful reiki sessions for me to understand that people make their own choices. Her pride was her worst enemy. Her pride took her life.

It started a few years ago. She had a few autoimmune diseases, but managed them with medication. Eventually her body started to wear out and she developed scarring on her lungs. She thought that these were just the cards she was dealt and learned to manage them without letting anyone think that anything was wrong. One day she decided to start losing weight, using her newfound free time in retirement to work on her physical appearance. It was very important to her. No one noticed as she began to waste away from a size 12 or size 14 to a size 00. I would ask her what she was doing and she would reply, "Cutting my portions back."

Food restriction is very dangerous, as you just read. Her malnourished and autoimmune diseased body grew weaker and weaker, so much so that she could barely stand up from a seated position. She wasn't an old woman. The whole family turned a blind eye because they were more focused on how good she looked. They encouraged the behavior with compliments. I knew better, but I have learned the lesson of not being a prophet in my own home. Regardless, I saw her waste away and could do nothing.

Eventually her body was far too susceptible to disease and she caught pneumonia and passed only a week after contracting it. She was unconscious when my family notified me, and by the time I arrived after flying all night, at her hospital room, at one in the morning- I could feel that her soul had already left us.

You see, body fat isn't always the enemy. It can actually act as a protecting layer when we need it the most. If we have zero body fat, we have no defense system. She had suffered with health issues for years, but the second she restricted her diet and lost all of her weight, it was too late. The damage was done. I miss her every day.

This, to say the least, was an insanely eye opening experience for me as a professional nutritionist because it underscored the kind of erroneous thinking that is so damaging in our culture. We are obsessed with weight loss over optimal health and wellbeing. We think disease is only controlled by products and prescription medication-instead of eating clean, real food.

The Lies Of The Weight Loss Industry

I worked in a weight-loss clinic as the nutrition specialist and the game they played is real. They hire young, impressionable women with no conscience, most of them are thin by default, and they are not healthy eaters. True story: I saw one bring McDonalds in for lunch one day. I also witnessed one of the already very thin managers go on the pregnancy hormone diet, cutting her calories to 500 per day. She said it was to test the product, but I knew better. She had a fairly severe case of body dysmorphic disorder and lived on all of the weight-loss programs, despite having a petite frame.

Weight-loss clinics want to hire ultrathin women as a constant reminder of something that is completely unattainable. Looking at them, we will begin to believe that thin is the only way we should look. And so, we buy more of their products. It's a technique called Stockholm syndrome. They "kidnap" our mind and then make us believe the lies they are telling us. This company called it neuro-linguistic programming (NLP), and it is a risky psych technique that falls dangerously close to brain-washing. They use posturing and tones to establish a comfortable dominance. Basically, they brainwash us into spending more money.

I have never used this crazy talk. I just got real with people and they respected me for it. I also never recommended anything I didn't believe in. I'm not a soulless, money-obsessed zombie. And if the job wasn't bad enough, coaches like me also had to weigh in monthly and have our body composition tested. Every month we had to send these numbers into corporate. We had to have 27 percent body fat or under, or else our job was on the line. Believe me, under was encouraged. We were highly encouraged, as already thin women, to go on the plans and to lose more weight. It seemed normal at the time, but now I understand how disgusting that was.

They are pimps and cheap car salesmen; they are not our friends. The women that work at these facilities have issues of their own and no business telling us that we are fat and unworthy. We don't need to lose weight, ever, unless we want to. The choice is always ours! We should want to strive to be HEALTHY, not SKINNY. Toxin build up or the body being in a diseased state, and not weight, is the only concern in my book. Whenever I gain fat tissue, it is due to eating or drinking too much sugar, in turn my estrogen increases, my body doesn't work very well, and my hormones get super messed up. This is my body, not yours, it is all a bioindividual experience. Everyone is different. Some of you have thyroid disorders, or other auto immune metabolic diseases. Focus on correcting your health, not losing weight.

What Holds You Back?

When a person is struggling with her food choices and ultimately her health, it is most likely due to a number of issues.

Trauma of any kind can affect a person negatively. Sometimes the issue is an unsatisfying job, unhealthy relationship, low self-worth, or an idea that she just isn't good enough. Sometimes women become unhealthy because of diagnosed or undiagnosed conditions. In most cases, the emotional trauma of any of these situations destroys the metabolism and the only control mechanism a person has left when presented with these situations is food.

Perhaps we feel as though we can't control what happens in our life, and at least food will bring us happiness, at least momentarily. We may feel as though we do everything in our power to change, and still our health is in decline. But why? Why do we emotionally eat, why can we still not find the answer to our health issues, and why are we ultimately unhappy? The truth is if we don't enter a place of growth, emotionally, we will never find the answers to these dilemmas. We will never fully understand how to make the right choice for our health. We will never be able to investigate the reality of personal health and how to unlock the answers to achieve optimal health and wellness if we don't first understand our emotions: who we are, what we need, how our body works, and what we need to nourish it.

Skinny Doesn't Mean Healthy

You may have found your salvation. You may have found a plan that keeps your weight down and keeps you in your "skinny" jeans, but you can't seem to fix that pesky digestive issue, or still have that auto-immune disease, or your skin never quite gets that dewy glow you always hear about. I hate to break it to you, but skinny doesn't always mean healthy.

I knew a woman once who was in charge of several weight-loss centers. She took medications for many issues including Hashimoto's hypothyroiditis, and had severe adrenal fatigue, to the point where she was borderline for having Addison's disease. Despite these warning signs she continued to diet and work out

7 days a week. Because she was thin, everyone thought she was healthy. Unfortunately she refused to listen to her body's many cries for help, due to her image. This woman made her money off of her image and not through representing real health. She was concerned with revenue and not the fact that the health of a lot of people on the program was being jeopardized. Remember, People are always watching and wondering what each other is doing. You can either set good example and inspire other to be healthy or you can do the exact opposite and be the destruction in another person's life. The products they sold were in my opinion, inedible, and most likely the cause of inflammation for most if not all the clients they sold them to. The cheap, processed, chemical ingredients in the supplements and foods they were forced to purchase were definitely jeopardizing their health. Women have become obsessed with the word "healthy." "Oh this food is good for me to eat because it's healthy." There is no such thing as a food being "healthy."

We, as a culture, desperately need precision of language. Food is only ever "nutrient dense" or "lacking in nutrient density." Weight-loss bars and supplement foods (with the exception of a very choice few) are typically anything but nutrient dense, therefore, not healthy for you at all. Why? Because you are not healthy after you eat them.

If your protein bar or frozen low-calorie meal has over five ingredients in it, and those ingredients aren't whole, organic, non-GMO, soy free, corn free, chemical and filler free, you shouldn't be eating it! It is not real food!

People might think they feel great because they lost sixty pounds doing some quick diet. Unfortunately, they have most likely caused more long-term damage to their body, and still didn't learn how to eat properly. Like I said before, and will say again, I'm not blaming anyone because we didn't know.

I'm sure the weight-loss expert seemed kind and determined. When desperation sets in we will try anything. We have tried everything and again, nothing has worked long term. We stay hopeful, thinking, this next one will be it, but sadly we are sold a pack of lies.

The idea that skinny automatically means healthy drives me absolutely crazy! One time, I was on a road trip for a wedding and my friend's mother proceeded to tell me that one of her friends was so fit and healthy, but had just gone through chemotherapy. It took everything inside of me not to have a meltdown and say, "Listen, your friend is anything but healthy. She just went through chemo, she had cancer! She's been sick. Just because she is skinny, doesn't mean she is healthy!" **Skinny does not equal healthy.**

Yes, we can sometimes lose weight when we are getting healthier, but this should not be our entire basis of measuring our overall health. We are going about it all wrong. Instead of focusing on health, we are stuck thinking about a number. Our weight on the scale is not the scale of health.

Let's imagine two women standing side by side. One is five-foot-six and weighs 120 pounds. People might think, by looking at her, that she is super healthy. Well, this woman also has active autoimmune diseases you can't see and takes several medications. The other woman is also five-foot-six and weighs 170 pounds. You think to yourself, "One hundred seventy pounds sounds like a lot for a five-six frame." Well, this second woman is a CrossFit® competitor, eats clean food, and takes no medications. She might have more body mass, but is actually the healthy one between the two women.

We are stuck on this idea that being thin magically equates to being healthy, but it is high time to put that falsehood in the trash and wake up to the truth. It's time to move forward into a new era and welcome the idea of real health. It's not about weight, it is so much more than that, it's about finding our HAPPY WEIGHT, it's about thriving, and being healthy.

NUTRITION IS NOT WHAT WE THOUGHT

Nutrition is something everyone thinks they have the answer to these days. Like I said earlier, people that think they know everything, most weight-loss experts or health coaches, are some of the most ignorant when it comes to real health. The sad part about discussing the effect of bad science is that it takes us half a century to realize we've made a mistake, and another half century to fix the current state of our nation's health. The science of healthy eating is an ever-evolving field and we have so many of the answers now. It's just up to us to spread the word and implement these healthy changes as quickly as we possibly can. Keeping up with the literature is the only way to know what is really happening. Paying close attention to the importance of Bioindividuality, bio specific macronutrient ratios, and clean eating is truly the way we should be approaching nutrition now. All of the low-calorie regimens, shakes, weight-loss supplements, quick fixes, and crash diets may help us lose weight for a hot minute, but we will quickly lose momentum if we come to rely on them and can create further issues with our health.

Crash diets help you cut weight, but what are you losing? Water and muscle? There are so many unhealthy body ratios out there because of fad diets. Cleanses can destroy your health. [6] I'm not a doctor so I can't legally say what you should or shouldn't do, but ask yourself: is your doctor telling you the truth?

I met a man once after teaching a corporate nutrition class and he asked me about the portion of the class that warned against doing cleanses or detoxes. He asked me, "Why did you say that cleanses are not safe?" I answered simply, "Because most people don't have the proper information. If the detoxification pathways in your organs aren't open and functioning, you could do serious harm to your systems that can lead to long-term damage." He then proceeded to tell me how he quickly developed a thyroid condition after doing repetitive weeklong water fasting, with complete food and beverage (other than water) restriction. This gentleman had no pre-existing thyroid complications until he started fasting. Also, thyroid conditions in men are not very common at all. So this really was detrimental to his health.

Here's a direct quote from Mario Skugor, M.D., an endocrinologist at the Cleveland Clinic: "Hypothyroidism is about eight to ten times less common in men. That's because 80 percent of hypothyroidism is caused by autoimmune disease, and autoimmune diseases are more common in women."[7]

The moral of the story is, you never know what could happen to you if you do a detox, cleanse, or any diet for that matter. Like I said, this one man believed he developed a serious metabolic autoimmune disease from fasting! Until you have all the facts about what works for your body as an individual, you shouldn't trust random advice.

Here are a few books you might want to read before being too trusting of random advice. *The Wahls Protocol* by Terry Wahls, *Grain Brain* by David Perlmutter, *The GAPS Diet* by Natasha Campbell McBride, *The Cholesterol Myths* by Uffe Ravnskov, *Why Stomach Acid is Good for You* by Johnathan Wright and Lane Lenard, *Nutrition and Physical Degeneration* by Weston A Price, and *Pottenger's Prophecy* by Grey Graham.

I get it, that's a lot of books to read. But above all, we are here on a journey to take control of our own health and stand in a space that is educated on the truth about our bodies. Right now, we don't have enough information, and we need a little enlightenment. We desperately need to take control of our health. We want a whole foundation, not a cracked one!

A CRACKED FOUNDATION

Let's take a visual approach to what I am trying to convey here. Imagine that your health is a concrete foundation. Are you taking any medications, either over the counter or prescribed? Do you have a diagnosed condition or disease? Do you have trouble sleeping, hormone imbalances, digestive issues, migraines, or allergies?

If any of these apply, then your foundation is cracked. The more the foundation cracks, the more the structure will begin to shift and fall apart. Diets and medications are only Band-Aid's, and you can't put Band-Aid's on a crack in your foundation. There needs to be a total understanding of your system, how it works, and how to rebuild that foundation from the ground up. You can't just pour concrete in it and expect it to get better.

What I am trying to say is that there is an underlying cause to any effect in the body. Even things that may seem normal like gas, bloating, or belching are not normal conditions. There is an underlying issue. But just as much as there is no one size fits all diet, there is no one size fits all approach to your body. Some of my readers may be thinking: *Then how the hell do I figure out what's going on with me?* The process is simple. We go north to south, and anything deeper than that requires further investigation with a holistic practitioner.

A HAPPY GUT

When you read this, you may think I'm crazy, but the integrity of the entire body's health is in the gut. Your gut is not only your second brain; it is also the driver of all major body processes. In the book by Natasha Campbell McBride, *The GAPS Diet,* she discusses the intensity of our body's microflora and how important the lining of our small intestines are. Have you ever heard of "leaky gut," or intestinal permeability? It's okay if you haven't, most people have not. *Leaky gut,* as nutritional therapists like to call it, is a condition in which an improper digestive mechanism causes the microvilli, the nutrient absorbers and intestine protectors, in the small intestines to retard, and then deteriorate the mucosal lining. This causes the intestinal wall to tear. When the holes are created, whole food passes directly into the blood stream, causing severe inflammation and for some, an autoimmune response.[8]

INFLAMMATORY FOOD IS CAUSING YOUR DISEASE

You see, if whole food passes into the blood stream, the body recognizes it as a foreign object. Antibodies are created, histamine levels are elevated, and the food is seen as an allergen or becomes a sensitivity. You'll see a lot of people develop food sensitivities at a later age due in large part to intestinal permeability, or leaky gut.[9] You may have discovered that you can't have gluten, dairy, or other foods. You just feel off and no one can give you an answer, except by shoving a new medication down your throat. The sad thing is that you know something is off, something isn't working properly, but you can't quite put your finger on it.

If you're like some people, you can't lose fat tissue because of a buildup of inflammation. It's not just a game of macronutrients vs. micronutrients, or portions, or calories. The body is so much more complicated than a numbers game, and inflammation is serious. Inflammation is at the root cause of almost all failures in the human body.

Did you know that some women have genetic liver congestion that causes estrogen dominance, making them more prone to have metabolic disorders and hormone imbalances? Estrogen not metabolizing properly in your liver or C-2 pathways can cause it to manifest in other negative and malignant ways, such as cancer.

Some women have such strong insulin resistance that if they merely look at a starch carbohydrate they gain fat tissue. And why is that? Because they don't have fully operating systems to breakdown starch and carbohydrates. Some women weren't born with the proper set of enzymes to digest basic foods groups like dairy proteins.

My point is that there are too many factors involved in digestion and weight gain, and that is why there is NO ONE SIZE FITS ALL approach.

INFLAMMATION IS THE ONLY COMMON DENOMINATOR

So what causes this inflammatory and autoimmune response? Good question!

Stress, processed food, packaged food, restaurant food, a lack of sleep, poor lifestyle habits, food sensitivities, alcohol, caffeine, medications, over-the-counter drugs, genetic mutations, or a gut that's poorly populated with beneficial microflora. The list goes on and on.

Because of one or more of these factors, we are having health issues, so how do we fix them? For some people, it will be simple and for others, it may take a while. Remember this is about bioindividuality and specific nutrition, not a quick fix! If we want sustainability we have to put the work in, there are no short cuts.

We begin with the north to south process (NTSP). This is a term I learned in school. I did not create or formulate this information, this is well developed and in practice all over the world. To understand the NTSP one must first get familiar with one's own body. The NTSP is the concept of digestion and body homeostasis relying completely on starting all health concerns from the beginning of the digestion process, the brain. Digestion begins in the brain, when we recognize food we begin to salivate.[10]

DIGESTION *Process*

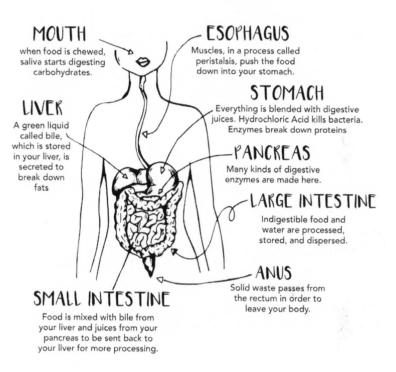

MOUTH
when food is chewed, saliva starts digesting carbohydrates.

ESOPHAGUS
Muscles, in a process called peristalsis, push the food down into your stomach.

STOMACH
Everything is blended with digestive juices. Hydrochloric Acid kills bacteria. Enzymes break down proteins

LIVER
A green liquid called bile, which is stored in your liver, is secreted to break down fats

PANCREAS
Many kinds of digestive enzymes are made here.

LARGE INTESTINE
Indigestible food and water are processed, stored, and dispersed.

ANUS
Solid waste passes from the rectum in order to leave your body.

SMALL INTESTINE
Food is mixed with bile from your liver and juices from your pancreas to be sent back to your liver for more processing.

DIGESTION

The body is positively fascinating. The main body parts involved are the mouth, the esophagus, the stomach, the duodenum, the liver, the gallbladder, the pancreas, the small and large intestines, the colon, and the rectum. That's a lot of body parts! Yeah, well, digestion is a big freaking deal. If food is used as medicine, then the digestive process better be intricate.

So now you know your body a little better. Let's go deeper. Remember when I said digestion begins in the brain? Yes, okay, well how exactly? The brain is our driver for response, correct?

Correct. So in order for the body to properly digest, the brain needs to get into a parasympathetic, or relaxed, state. Once that is achieved, the sight and smell of food causes the brain to send signals to the mouth where the cheeks begin to salivate, causing the stomach to stimulate gastric juice production. Every process is crucial, and saliva is a big deal. Without salivary amylase we are not able to start the breakdown of carbohydrates, including fruits & vegetables. Once our saliva is enacted we begin to chew. Chewing, or mastication, is HUGE! If we do not properly chew our food, imagine how much harder our body has to work to break food down.

Slow Down

If we eat really fast or rarely chew our food and we have digestive issues, speed may be a primary contributing factor. Slow down, chew your food!! The next step in the process is swallowing the bolus, or food ball. Once we have swallowed the food it travels down the esophagus to the stomach. The gastric juices, Hydrochloric Acid (HCL) and Pepsinogen, have already been triggered to release. These juices are essential for protein break down.

You may have heard that red meat is bad for you because it takes too long to digest, right? You may actually have a sensitivity to specific red meats. I have seen allergies to all different kinds of food. Or perhaps, you just don't have enough acid in your stomach. Have you ever eaten a steak and had a stomach ache afterwards? Steak is pure muscle meat, and if you don't have adequate HCL in your stomach you will have a hard time breaking that protein down. Make sense?

Our food has now hopefully turned into chyme, or just a pool of food juice. If not, we will continue to experience gastric discomfort, among other issues such as acid reflux, constipation, and diarrhea. Once the chyme passes through the duodenum, enzymes are released from the pancreas, liver, and gallbladder to process fats and glucose. Ninety percent of nutrient absorption will happen in the small intestines.

The chyme will continue to travel through the large intestines and colon. Right before the exit point, excess water, as well as fat soluble vitamins A, D, E, and K will be absorbed into our system. If we experience irritable bowel syndrome (IBS), Crohn's disease, or colitis, these essential vitamins will be the most depleted. That can make it hard to fully function or have a healthy immune system, leaving us feeling constantly weak and ill.

I think you get the gist of digestion now, right? It's very complicated and needs to be paid close attention to. If you get an upset stomach after you eat and do not have healthy, regular bowel movements every day, you are in a diseased state!

Let's back up to leaky gut causing damage to our system. There is obviously a crack in our foundation somewhere, and there can be a number of issues as a result. This is where bioindividuality comes in.

Every single person on this planet is different, with a different genetic makeup, different microbiome diversity (gut bacteria), different lifestyle habits and choices, different environments, and different stresses and reactions to them. We all have so many avenues to explain why we are where we are with our health. This is exactly why it is so important to understand that there is no one right answer that will work for everyone. We have to understand our body and what it is capable of, before we can say, "This is it. This is what worked for me."

Epigenetics And Gene Expression

To one degree or another, we all know what genes are, right? They are the tiny, but complicated, bits and pieces that make up who we are as individuals. Some of us have genetic predispositions, and some of us don't. Let us discuss in the easiest way possible, the difference between genetic expression and epigenetics.

Gene expression is a tightly regulated process that allows a cell to respond to its changing environment. In layman's terms, this is when a bad gene can be "turned on" by poor lifestyle and diet habits. Just as much as a gene can be "turned on," it can also be "turned off." When turned off, the person has reduced the inflammatory response by diet and lifestyle changes and the gene no longer needs to be expressed, therefore reversing the negative signs and symptoms.

People often believe they are doomed to certain health outcomes. I often hear, "My mother died from breast cancer, so I'm likely next." Not necessarily. If that person chooses to make different lifestyle and diet choices, they may be able to avoid the disease all together by keeping their gene in the "off" position, or dormant, permanently.

This however, does not mean that those without the genetic predisposition are in the clear, which brings us to epigenetics. Epigenetics is the process by which genetic codes can be rewritten by poor diet and lifestyle habits, but only expressed in offspring and future generations. Meaning, if a person decides to take horrible care of her body and then has children, those children will be worse off than she was. I have seen so many women eat terribly before, during, and after pregnancy and then claim that they have no idea why their children are so sick or have so many allergies, because they never did. "You are what you eat" could not ring more true in this moment.

If a parent has a high inflammatory response before a child is born, she will likely rewrite the child's genetic code while stripping the child of healthy gut bacteria, and pass on to the child a weakened immune system or worse, developmental delays.

Is this a death sentence for all? Are our culture's epigenetics a doomsday prophecy? Can genes be "turned off" if they are already being expressed? That all depends on what you are willing to do and how badly you want to focus solely on your health and not your image. Everyone is capable of change.

Here is how I found my way to changing my eating habits

and drastically altering my lifestyle. Let's start with a series of personal accounts and experiences I have had throughout my time in nutrition therapy.

My History With Food Sensitivities

As a child I had no idea what was good for me, what I was sensitive to, and what made me feel sick. All I knew was that I was sick after every meal. I thought it was normal, I thought that was what life was like. I also didn't know that I couldn't pay attention in school because the food I was eating all day, every day, was poisoning me. I never had energy to be active. I couldn't understand how everyone around me was simply good at everything they did, and why life was such a struggle for me. I had horrible allergies, sneezing all day. Horrible acne covered my body. I wore a lot of perfume and deodorant to cover up my body odor. Bad body odor is caused by a detoxing or toxic liver. I had no way of knowing that my poor liver was always in detox mode from all of the inflammatory foods I was eating.

As I entered adulthood, I finally had a blood test done. Not voluntarily. It wasn't an "I should do this" kind of moment. It was something I ate that helped me get there. I had eaten a Subway wrap and had a horrible allergic reaction to the tomato inside. Up to this point, I had never eaten a raw tomato. Any tomato I ate was in the form of high-fructose corn syrup in ketchup or overly processed, nonperishable salsa. Organic foods should never be "nonperishable." So, I ate this fresh tomato and called my mom freaking out that my breath was labored and I was itching intensely everywhere. She instructed that I take a Benadryl and that next time I was home from college I should get a blood test done. So I did. I am not saying taking Benadryl is okay, because it's not. It is a Band-Aid, but sometimes a necessary one when we are in panic mode.

It Wasn't All In My Head

The results were fairly shocking. My blood tested positive for sensitivity to wheat, rice, potato, tomato, corn, and soy. It all made sense as to why I was getting migraines after drinking my soy lattes. I didn't just wake up one day and say, "Eureka! I think I'll change the way I eat!" There is always a cause, a starting point, and a reason. Things have to get so bad that we actually pay attention. It sounds messed up, but that is American society today. We honestly believe that everything we are doing, and everything we have been taught is right and the answer to our health problems.

It took another ten years until I made the choice to give up wheat for good. You see, I made every excuse in the book as to why I could eat wheat occasionally, until I couldn't. I developed a pretty severe case of leaky gut that depleted my nutrients so drastically that it altered my microflora and caused debilitating anxiety, suicidal depression, heart palpitations, and bouts of paranoia. I am not a huge fan of alarming people, so no one knew except for my now husband, a few close friends, and a few choice family members. Honestly, I look back at it now and think that I am grateful for the experience. I have learned to be super in tune with my body, mindful of all the choices I make, and extremely proactive when I feel as though something is off.

What worked for my body to reverse these conditions? Some things that may or may not work for you, but this is what worked for me:

I removed all gluten from my daily life, forever. Gluten and I broke up; we have gone our separate ways. I removed any and all chemically processed foods: no preservatives, no dyes, no additives, no hidden ingredients, no fillers, no non-organics, no GMOs, except bananas, which are all genetically modified. All of my meat and eggs are 100 percent grass-fed, pasture raised, and uncured. I care about sustainability and where my food comes from. I basically stopped eating the crap we see on TV and the crap we find in conventional grocery stores. I stopped shopping in the aisles and only shopped the perimeter. This means that I eat fresh foods and real foods, all foods my body can digest.

I also drink bone broth, and eat liver. I eat foods with live, active cultures in them, like raw, fermented sauerkraut and pickles. When I am eating dairy, I consume only 100 percent grass-fed dairy products.

I dramatically increased my fat intake, and removed all hydrogenated vegetable oils like canola oil. I make sure that fats like canola oil and margarine never touch my food. I basically threw out anything in my house that was a chemical dump. The only oils I have in my house now are 100 percent grass-fed ghee and butter, unfiltered 100 percent organic non-GMO coconut oil, pasture-raised duck fat, grass-fed tallow (cow fat), and pasture-raised lard (pig fat).

Yes, I eat animal fats, a lot of animal fats, and my cholesterol level is amazing. I don't gain fat tissue from eating fat.

No, I am not genetically gifted. This is the way some of us are meant to eat. Like eating fat. Fat is essential for women. It is imperative to consume fat for our cells to rejuvenate and to communicate with each other. Thankfully, recent studies have debunked the cholesterol myths. Dietary cholesterol has absolutely zero effect on your body's cholesterol. Inflammation is the root cause of bad cholesterol, and causes of inflammation are different in every person. But it is not caused by consuming animal fats. Heart disease has nothing to do with dietary cholesterol. This is not a joke.

THE TRUTH ABOUT FATS

A 2014 *Time Magazine* article detailing the ways in which physicians were wrong about fat and how imperative it is to our health was such a breath of fresh air.[11] Finally, the truth about nutrition comes out and it turns out that fat was never bad for you. Fat is essential for daily life and the integrity of health in the human body. Saturated fat, the most important and healthiest fat is directly responsible for cell-to-cell communication and hormone production. I am probably blowing your mind right now, and you are in utter disbelief and hope I'm joking. But please, refer to the previous books or article listed and then we can discuss disbelief. I would never lead you astray.

Take special note of the book written by Terry Wahls, M.D., a woman whose multiple sclerosis (MS) was so severe that she became disabled and relied on a gravity chair for over eight years. Through the miracle of eating whole, nutrient-dense foods with the right macronutrients and adding healthy fats, plus practicing meditation and using electric stimulation, Dr. Wahls was able to reverse an "irreversible" disease and can now not only walk, but ride a bike, and run. She accomplished this without the help of pharmaceutical drugs and without new age miracle treatment. She did it with food and copious amount of fat![12]

Of course, all of this is a process; she didn't just wake up one day and have all of the answers. That's why happy weight is a state of being. Her discovery of her bioindividuality was like the process that most women go through when making huge strides in their wellness goals. I am sure she went through a process like I describe in this book: confidence, vulnerability, saying no, finding her tribe, and breaking up with foods.

Will her exact plan: a sulfur rich, keto-paleo protocol with transcendental meditation, work for you? It depends. That's the beauty of bioindividuality: it all depends on what your genetics are, what current issues you have, if you have food allergies or leaky gut. Do you have a parasite or bacterial overgrowth? Do you have metal toxicity or nutrient deficiencies? One size never fits all. This is why happy weight is the anti-diet and why I am here to share a message with you about finding what works for your body and your body alone!

Let's discuss the possibilities of what could be happening in your body, how to find out the truth, and where to go from there.

Our Bodies Are Complicated

Are we in agreement now that what we thought we knew to be true is not? Our bodies are so incredibly complicated, there are so many contributing factors, and we are all so different. The diet that works for "Amy" will not work for "Jill", and vice versa. Lifestyle and genetics are huge factors. Nora Gedgaudas, author of *Primal Body, Primal Mind,* states that genetics are like a loaded gun and our diet pulls the trigger.[13] Remember back to gene expression? Let's recap: It means we can turn a gene on and off with diet and lifestyle. The tricky part is that since lifestyle and diet can turn a gene on, genetic mutations across a population become more likely.

Let's use another example: if we have the arthritis gene, that doesn't mean we will automatically get arthritis, though we are more susceptible to it. It means that if we are not careful with diet and lifestyle choices, the gene will "turn on," and we will suffer the symptoms of this autoimmune disease.

Now on the flip side, a gene can be "turned off," meaning we can reverse the symptoms if we correct the inflammatory cause. Just like we learned in science class as children, Newton's third law of motion applies: With every action there is an equal and opposite reaction.[14] Genetic predisposition is in no way a death sentence; it's a warning sign. It's up to us if we chose to listen to the cautionary tale or not. Life is always about choices. Which do we choose? What action will we take?

So You Thought Your Diet Worked

When they arrive, most of my clients have been following a low-fat diet or anti-red meat diet most of their lives and think that they have had great success with it in the past. Are you the same? Well, maybe you did have success, but the success was most likely only due to a calorie deficit, not a fat or red meat deficit. It is entirely possible that some of the issues you have with your health today are directly related to the absence of fat or proper proteins in your diet. However, there are some who know that saturated fat is good for you and congratulations to them! But you are reading this book for a reason and may not be paying attention to the deeper attributes of a complete holistic lifestyle to avoid a diseased state.

Death By Food Pyramid

Let's look at how we got here, what changed in our diets, and how health in America became the laughing stock of the rest of the planet. Studies help with disbelief and intense scrutiny of health proclamations, so here's another book. *Death by Food Pyramid* is an amazing book written by Denise Minger.[16] Minger is not a household name, but she should be. She is one of the few females in our modern day medical history that has completely disproved the USDA food guidelines and pyramid chart (too many grains and bad fats), the China Study (a predominantly plant based diet, high in soy products)[16], and the Seven Countries Study (red meat is bad)[17]. You haven't heard of her because her studies make her wildly unpopular with the people who make millions of dollars off of those fad diets. She points out how this way of eating is killing us and why grains are the worst things being perpetuated in agriculture today. We are at a pinnacle of innovation and technological genius. So why are we still so ignorant when it comes to what is healthy and what isn't?

The answer is money. Have you ever heard of Monsanto? ConAgra? No? Well, they're powerful agribusinesses that use their considerable wealth to lobby governments around the world and control the flow of information about the food supply. We need to understand why food today is not what it once was, and this is a major factor.

How Our Food Changed

World War II changed everything, in more ways than one. Food was one of the most significant changes. We needed to find a way to store and preserve food for our troops, so the canning industry was born. What canned soup was in the beginning and what is has become are two polar opposites, like most packaged and processed foods today. Canned food in the beginning, over sixty years ago, wasn't that bad. Then corporations saw an opportunity to make more money with mass shipping and production. We became a supply and demand culture that was created by our massive growth, and the ad agencies responsible for selling the idea were geniuses. Placating our every desire and the promise of a better tomorrow is what we think we are buying when we go the grocery store. The truth is, today, we are buying cheap crap with endless chemicals and fillers.

Our food supply no longer resembles the truth and happiness of times past. Many of us nutrition professionals call it a chemical shit storm. These foods are made in factory farms, injected with antibiotics and hormones, with animals that have no room to breathe. It is an agricultural hell dripping in glyphosate, a liquid poison, staffed by workers wearing Hazmat suits, working in processing plants with multiple outputs, causing cross contamination. If we think the food we are eating is safe because we heated it or washed it, we are just continuing the belief that has been spoon fed to us by the media driven and money hungry food & beverage industries.

DEATH BY DENATURED FOODS

The moment the animal we are eating is fed grain and confined, it becomes diseased. Why does the American Medical Association tell us a meatless diet is best?[18] Because the meat we are eating isn't good for us. Am I promoting vegetarianism? No. I am promoting quality and education. Animal fats and proteins are necessary for human life; we just need to know what kind to eat, and where they should come from. Are there healthy vegans and vegetarians? Yes, if they are doing it correctly, but that is not the answer for everyone. Remember what I said before, **one size never fits all!**

Francis Pottenger, Jr., M.D., was an amazing scientist that did a controlled study on the effects of living organisms consuming denatured (chemically processed) foods. A denatured food is the deconstruction of a foods naturally occurring protein or enzyme. Protein and enzyme structure can alter in meat, dairy, and eggs, when the animal is fed a diet that is not according to their natural state.[19]

The end game is that you will become what your food eats if you do not seek out viable food sources and consume animal proteins in their natural state- like grass fed beef, pasture raised poultry, grass fed and raw dairy, and organic vegetables and fruits.

To find out what works for you, you need to get at the root causes of any disease or discomfort you're feeling and what makes you ultimately unhealthy. Some folks out there have incredible metabolisms and are able to eat whatever they want and not gain an ounce. Others can smoke cigarettes and drink whiskey every day and live to be one hundred. This is the wonderful dance of genetics, a beautiful collection of gut bacteria, a positive emotional environment, and the lack of inflammation.

As you may or may not have guessed, inflammation is the root cause of all disease on a cellular level. Inflammation is caused by a few different factors. It's crazy to think that the food we have been eating all of our lives is what has predominately contributed to our diabetes, cancer, hypothyroidism, gallbladder disease and so on. But this is 100 percent correct.

Like I mentioned before, I have had food sensitivities my entire life. No one knew what was wrong with me, it wasn't a thing we thought about back then, unless you had a peanut allergy or were lactose intolerant. When I got the gastritis diagnosis and was always nauseous, gassy, bloated, or had a headache after I ate, it was hilariously, just the food I was eating. I could never focus in school and had little to no energy. When I was prescribed the six sets of antibiotics like I explained earlier, the antibiotics didn't work, so the next step for my doctor was surgery. I see this time and time again, when doctors are unsuccessful with drugs, they perform expensive and sometimes unnecessary surgery. My doctor performed a major surgery to remove my tonsils, adenoids, nasal polyps, and correction of a collapsed nostril.

Because I am allergic to opioids, I could only take ibuprofen before and after the surgery, which caused me serious intestinal damage, led to leaky gut, and pushed me into severe anxiety and depression by my mid-twenties. My anxiety got so bad that at one point I was deathly afraid of flying and felt uncomfortable even riding in cars with other people, due to the fear that I was going to die. This is not normal. Even though millions of Americans suffer from anxiety and depression, it is not normal! Not only is it not normal, the psyche diagnosis most receive, they stop there. Most people don't understand that brain chemicals are controlled by our gut health. We can change our mood and behavior with diet and diet alone, we don't always need the interference of prescription medication. You can get better, you just need to investigate what will work for you!

With the help of eating real, whole, nutrient-dense foods and supplementing them with the nutrients my body was seriously lacking, like vitamin D, amino acids, minerals, fats, protein, and so on, I was able to completely change all of that. Finding out what foods work for my body forever changed my life.

It is so powerful and amazing to know that food can be used as medicine. All I had to do was remove one major food group--in my case, anything with gluten in it. Your good foods and bad foods will be different than mine. It is high time you look at the foods that cause you inflammation, as you might want to give them up. No excuses. It could be gluten, or dairy, or eggs, or nightshades (tomatoes and potatoes). Everyone is different. What causes you to react?

How do you even know if you have a food sensitivity? That's a whole other question in itself. If you feel excessive fullness after meals, get bloated, or gassy, you are 100 percent sensitive to something and have a lack of viable gastric juices to break that food down. Some people start taking digestive enzymes because they are not emotionally prepared to deal with the truth, which is: it's time to give up the food that hurts them!

I have personal experience with this exact struggle. These words aren't coming from a negative place, or as a result of my being a nutritionist. Breaking up with gluten was one of the hardest things I have ever done, and now five years off gluten, I have seen the other side and will never go back. A lot of gluten-free eaters make exceptions and say, "Only a little here and there." But unfortunately, the body doesn't work like that. The little bits here and there may not deliver an immediate reaction, but the inflammation will develop over time on a foundational level. These little bits can eventually destroy the immune system. Think of a dam in a river, if you poke tiny holes, eventually over time that dam will collapse.

Most people live to eat and do not eat to live. The mentality in America is overabundance. We supersize everything like we think we are going to starve, and we are obsessed with our particular brand of something, saying, "I'm a Pepsi drinker" or "I follow the South Beach diet" or "I'm a foodie, I can't cut foods out." American-style marketing is genius and we have become people that identify with our brand of food or product. If we identify with anything other than eating real food, that's where we are getting it wrong.

We as a nation, desperately need to give up the foods that keep us from being healthy, bottom line. It's so sad to see my lactose-intolerant friends still eat dairy even though it causes severe intestinal discomfort or other inflammatory responses, just because it tastes good.

Food sensitivities are some of the top causes of inflammation. Remember that inflammation is at the root cause of disease. So yes, your food sensitivity is and always will be a large contributing factor to inhibiting your health recovery, achieving your happy weight, decreasing your arthritis symptoms, stopping your bladder or yeast infections, reversing your thyroid condition, or reversing your PCOS (poly cystic ovarian syndrome). The list goes on and on.

Let's discuss for a moment how food, lifestyle, and environment can contribute to fat tissue gain, so that we can begin to understand how all of this is connected. Remember, one size never fits all. Every single person is different and we each gain fat tissue for different reasons, and struggle with losing that fat tissue for different reasons. The following is going to be a very simple anatomy and physiology lesson with some nutrition added to understand how the natural processes work.

I want you to walk away knowing that there is a right answer for everyone, but you will have to make the choice on your own. I will also discuss briefly the anomalies and difficult cases I have seen, and how I figured them out.

Here is one example of a reason we become unhealthy. Let's say that we have no known autoimmune disorder or endocrine issues, and are seemingly "healthy," but we can't seem to achieve our happy weight. We regularly consume processed foods at home and eat out the rest of the time. These processed foods are devoid of nutrients, meaning there is no nutritional value. No, frozen diet food in a box is not healthy, because it's not even real food.

Digestion Is Imperitive

It begins with gastric juices. If you have ever experienced acid reflux, heartburn, gerd (gastroesophageal reflux disease), gas, or bloating, your stomach acid could be insufficient. Doctors like to tell us we have too much stomach acid and they put us on over the counter antacids. This is mainly the result of good marketing done by the pharmaceutical companies. HCL is something I will say again and again until you understand how important it is. The truth is you may have what we in the nutrition world like to call hypochlorhydria; an insufficient supply of HCL. Your body has created this issue by eating too many processed foods and being overly stressed and not mindful. Consuming excessive processed GMO carbohydrates, sugar, and overworking the body and mind are all contributing factors. When we have reached a non-homeostatic point in the body it will naturally begin to lack production in vital nutrients or acids. After the lack of HCL sets in and you can no longer digest food properly, these processed foods begin to cause systemic inflammation and paralysis of the microvilli, not to mention completely altering the gut micro-flora. Like I described earlier, the microvilli are in place to protect the intestinal lining, but overconsumption of processed foods has retarded the microvilli, causing intestinal permeability or a leaky gut.

Now you know that leaky gut syndrome is when a series of small holes in the intestinal lining allows undigested foods to pass directly into the blood stream, polluting the body. Once these undigested foods are in the blood they are seen as foreign invaders. The body then develops antibodies to deal with these foreign invaders, creating a histamine reaction, which is what most call an allergic reaction or food sensitivity. You can go through life without ever suffering from food sensitivities and wake up one day with a whole list of them.

Naturally, any of the foods you develop a sensitivity to will cause further inflammation all over the body. This inflammation, along with other processed foods you have been consuming, begins to toxify the liver. Double inflammation.

When the liver has reached a point that it can no longer process what we are ingesting or detoxify properly, insulin levels will cause overuse of cortisol. Cortisol loves to hold onto adipose tissue, or body fat. Cortisol is a stress hormone that helps our nervous system react to stressful situations. From an evolutionary standpoint, it developed to help us fight against environmental dangers like oversized animals. Lions, and tigers, and bears, oh my.

We have created an inflammatory response with the foods we are eating. This natural fight-or-flight hormone mechanism that lives in our adrenal glands will hold onto fat in any stressful, inflamed state. It is called "starvation mode." The body goes into starvation mode when we have too much stress. This stress is caused not only by the damage done to the digestive tract, but can also commonly be caused by physical and emotional stress.

This is why we see increases in weight after traumatic events. The overuse of cortisol can destroy our metabolism.

Do you have more food cravings during stressful events? I know that I certainly do. When we have excessive output of cortisol, the body will naturally crave salty, crunchy foods. When our glucose or thyroid levels are unbalanced, we tend to crave sweets. This is a natural process in the body that tells us things are out of control.

Stress is not a green light to give into our cravings and emotional discomfort and binge on whatever we want. It is the instruction to be mindful of what is happening inside our delicate system and react with nutrient-dense foods to correct the imbalance. Here is an amazing chart that talks about cravings and what to eat instead.[20]

This chart is so very important in part because, it helps us enter a place of true mindfulness when it comes to listening to our body. If we tap into our body's innate intelligence and listen oh so very carefully, we can eventually enter a place where we can truly understand what our body needs and how to nourish it. This exercise of "body talk" makes us ultimately more in tune with our body's systems their subtle alarms. I have reached a point in my life where now I can pin point even down to the very mineral my body is lacking. This act of mindfulness in listening to one's body is not only an amazing way to love your body, but also a relief to always wondering what the heck is going on. When you listen, you will know better than anyone. This is your body, no one else's. It's time to pay attention.

THE FOOD CRAVING CHART

IF YOU CRAVE THIS...	WHAT YOU REALLY NEED IS THIS...	AND HERE ARE HEALTHY FOODS THAT HAVE IT...
CHOCOLATE	MAGNESIUM	RAW NUTS AND SEEDS, LEGUMES, FRUITS
SWEETS	CHROMIUM	BROCCOLI, GRAPES, CHEESE, DRIED BEANS, CALVES LIVER, CHICKEN
	CARBON	FRESH FRUITS
	PHOSPHORUS	CHICKEN, BEEF LIVER, POULTRY, FISH, EGGS, DAIRY, NUTS, LEGUMES, GRAINS
	SULFUR	CRANBERRIES, HORSERADISH, CRUCIFEROUS VEGETABLES, KALE, CABBAGE
	TRYPTOPHAN	CHEESE, LIVER, LAMB, RAISINS, SWEET POTATO, SPINACH
BREAD/TOAST	NITROGEN	HIGH PROTEIN FOODS: FISH, MEAT, NUTS, BEANS
OILY SNACKS, FATTY FOODS	CALCIUM	MUSTARD AND TURNIP GREENS, BROCCOLI, KALE, LEGUMES, CHEESE, SESAME
COFFEE OR TEA	PHOSPHORUS	CHICKEN, BEEF, LIVER, POULTRY, FISH, EGGS, DAIRY, NUTS, LEGUMES
	SULFUR	EGG YOLKS, RED PEPPERS, MUSCLE PROTEIN, GARLIC, ONION, CRUCIFEROUS VEGETABLES
	SALT	SEA SALT, APPLE CIDER VINEGAR (ON SALAD)
	IRON	MEAT, FISH AND POULTRY, SEAWEED, GREENS, BLACK CHERRIES
ALCOHOL, RECREATIONAL DRUGS	PROTEIN	MEAT, POULTRY, SEAFOOD, DAIRY, NUTS
	AVENIN	GRANOLA, OATMEAL
	CALCIUM	MUSTARD AND TURNIP GREENS, BROCCOLI, KALE, LEGUMES, CHEESE, SESAME
	GLUTAMINE	SUPPLEMENT GLUTAMINE POWDER FOR WITHDRAWAL, RAW CABBAGE JUICE
	POTASSIUM	SUN–DRIED BLACK OLIVES, POTATO PEEL BROTH, SEAWEED, BITTER GREENS
CHEWING ICE	IRON	MEAT, FISH, POULTRY, SEAWEED, GREENS, BLACK CHERRIES
BURNED FOOD	CARBON	FRESH FRUITS
SODA	CALCIUM	MUSTARD AND TURNIP GREENS, BROCCOLI, KALE, LEGUMES, CHEESE, SESAME
SALTY FOODS	CHLORIDE	RAW GOAT MILK, FISH, UNREFINED SEA SALT
ACID FOODS	MAGNESIUM	RAW NUTS AND SEEDS, LEGUMES, FRUITS
PREFERENCE FOR LIQUIDS RATHER THAN SOLIDS	WATER	FLAVOR WATER WITH LEMON OR LIME. YOU NEED 8 TO 10 GLASSES PER DAY.
PREFERENCE FOR SOLIDS RATHER THAN LIQUIDS	WATER	FLAVOR WATER WITH LEMON OR LIME.
COOL DRINKS	MANGANESE	WALNUTS, ALMONDS, PECANS, PINEAPPLE, BLUEBERRIES
PMS CRAVINGS	ZINC	RED MEATS (ESPECIALLY ORGAN MEATS), SEAFOOD, LEAFY VEGETABLES, ROOT VEGETABLES
GENERAL OVEREATING	SILICON	NUTS, SEEDS; AVOID REFINED STARCHES
	TRYPTOPHAN	CHEESE, LIVER, LAMB, RAISINS, SWEET POTATO, SPINACH
	TYROSINE	VITAMIN C SUPPLEMENTS OR ORANGE, GREEN, RED FRUITS AND VEGETABLES
LACK OF APPETITE	VITAMIN B1	NUTS, SEEDS, BEANS, LIVER AND OTHER ORGAN MEATS
	VITAMIN B3	TUNA, HALIBUT, BEEF, CHICKEN, TURKEY, PORK, SEEDS AND LEGUMES
	MANGANESE	WALNUTS, ALMONDS, PECANS, PINEAPPLE, BLUEBERRIES
	CHLORIDE	RAW GOAT MILK, UNREFINED SEA SALT
TOBACCO	SILICON	NUTS, SEEDS; AVOID REFINED STARCHES
	TYROSINE	VITAMIN C SUPPLEMENTS OR ORANGE, GREEN AND RED FRUITS AND VEGETABLES

We have already gotten fairly technical here, but in short, stress will destroy every aspect of our body and will cause us to become unhealthy due to an excessive intake of unhealthy foods and a disrupted system. Health is not about calories; it's about nutrient density. Health is not about calorie restriction; it is about making sure every aspect of our internal health is sound. Mind, Body, Soul.

Do you have healthy digestion? Digestion is key when it comes to your health, but simply going to the bathroom every day is not the signifier of perfect health. On the next page is a poop chart to help you understand that pooping is an essential litmus test for your health.[21]

If you are not pooping properly, and you are experiencing any of the previous digestive issues I have brought up, your body is not healthy. It's time to clean up your choices, be aware that you are having health issues, and either break up with processed food or the foods that are causing you harm.

For those of you unable to absorb or process certain foods properly, you must understand the importance of how digestion works. The truth is in your poop. Your poop will tell you every time you go to the bathroom, how your body is responding to your eating and lifestyle choices.

Start with understanding and admitting that there is a problem and go from there.

HOW WELL DO YOU KNOW YOUR SHIT?

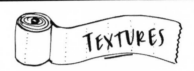

SEPARATE HARD LUMPS

You're lacking fiber & fluids. Drink more water & eat some fruits & veggies.

SAUSAGE SHAPED WITH SURFACE CRACKS

This is normal, but the cracks mean you could use more water.

SOFT BLOBS WITH CLEAR-CUT EDGES

Pretty normal if you're pooping multiple times.

SAUSAGE SHAPED, SMOOTH AND SOFT

optimal poop! you're fine!

SAUSAGE SHAPED BUT LUMPY

Not as serious as separate hard lumps, but you need to load up on fluids and fiber.

SOFT AND STICKS TO THE SIDES OF THE TOILET

Presence of too much oil, which could mean that your body isn't absorbing fats properly.

WATERY

You have diarrhea! This is probably caused by some sort of infection and diarrhea is your body's way of cleaning it out. Drink lots of liquids!

FLUFFY PIECES, MUSHY STOOL

On the edge of normal. This is on its way to becoming diarrhea.

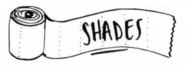

BROWN

You're fine. Poop is naturally brown.

BLACK

Could mean internal bleeding due to ulcer or cancer. Some vitamins can cause black poop too. Pay attention if it's sticky.

GREEN

Food may be moving through your large intestine too quickly. Or you could have eated lots of green veggies.

LIGHT WHITE OR CLAY-COLORED

If it's not what you're normally seeing, it could mean a bile duct obstruction. See a doc.

YELLOW

Greasy, foul-smelling yellow poop indicates excess fat.

RED OR BLOODY

Blood in your poop could be a symptom of cancer. Always see a doctor right away.

*Side note if your stool is red or seemingly bloody, make sure you didn't just eat beets.

The Not So Secret Life Of Your Gut Bacteria And Digestion

The human gut microbiome is fabulously complicated, so much so that experts are still researching it to understand how it works. Our gut bacteria are responsible for most of our major body processes and are typically where all diseases begin. If we do not have adequate gut bacteria or an optimally functioning digestive tract, we are often left with a system that will be driven to an inflammatory state.

Most belly fat or adipose tissue development is caused by a problem in one digestive organ or another. The pancreas is responsible for our insulin production; if that process is disrupted we can become extremely carb sensitive, making it very difficult for the body to properly digest starch carbohydrates. If we throw a kink into our insulin production and create resistance, then we can end up building quite an abundant amount of estrogen toxicity in our liver, another vital organ in the scope of our digestion and bacteria. This will inevitably affect the endocrine system, resulting in adrenal fatigue, causing over production in the stress hormone: cortisol. Belly fat is the direct result of stress and inflammation, which then transfers to the rest of the digestive system, and more importantly, the liver.

If the liver is filled with toxins, we will not be able to filter through the important material, causing a pretty serious hormone imbalance. If the liver is congested, the gallbladder will start to forget to do its job.

If we lose the optimal function of the gallbladder, we won't be able to process the proper healthy fats and dietary cholesterol that the body needs in order to engage hormone communication and cell regeneration, thus increasing cell retardation and inflammation. Side note: If you no longer have a gallbladder I highly recommend researching Bile Salts, they could save your life.

So what does all of this have to do with gut bacteria? Everything. If we do not digest with optimal organ function, we will be left with toxic waste buildup and inconsistent movements, and some of us will lose all motility and experience severe IBS or constipation. Some people walk around with up to fifteen pounds of un-eliminated fecal matter.[22] Yes, people can be literally full of shit.

This entire experience will elevate blood glucose levels, cause nutrient deficiency or malabsorption, leaky gut, estrogen dominance, fatty liver, intestinal disorders, and what people in my circle call *cortisol belly.*

Any number of the aforementioned issues could be the culprit. I find that when my clients get their gut in check and focus on stress reduction, that area tends to deflate and become less swollen.

Alcohol doesn't help this area at all. If you mess with your gut bacteria in a bad way, you will pay the price. Your gut bacteria is essential for optimal living and a healthy body overall.

So how do we help out the gut? There are so many ways. As we have discussed in extensive detail so far, every person's body and system are very different.

Some people take antibiotics like they are candy and most likely have a horrible yeast overgrowth in their intestines that causes them to crave carbs and sugar all day long. Others may have been born with a faulty system and need the GAPS protocol or something similar to get them back on track.

The truth in all of this is that you need to investigate. You will never become responsible for your own health if you don't take matters into your own hands.

One thing that has been a sure-fire way to begin for my clients and colleagues is to remove the crap from their diet:

highly processed oils such as canola, vegetable, margarine, and grapeseed, GMO foods, highly processed foods with more than five ingredients, dairy that isn't grass-fed or raw (highly processed, ultra-pasteurized dairy can be super inflammatory), and nonorganic produce.

Basically, stop eating junk. If you are not eating foods made from scratch, and everything comes from a package, it won't work.

Remove **Nightshades**! All tomatoes, peppers, potato's (not sweet potato's), and eggplant. These foods are highly inflammatory for most all people with pain, inflammatory or auto immune conditions.

Next, integrate some deliciously fermented foods like raw fermented sauerkraut, pickles, kombucha, or kimchee. These foods must be found in the refrigerated section, as true fermented foods are never in the dry goods section. In order to help your gut, the bacteria need to be alive and flourishing.

Probiotic supplements are always a good choice!

What works for you may not work for someone else, so try some and see what works for your body. The answer to all supplements or food protocols working is "it depends." There are no guarantees that what your friend is trying will work for you, remember: one size never fits all.

Nourishing Bone Broth Will Change Your Life

Bone broth has been a part of healing for centuries, since the beginning of civilization really. You can find bone broth in almost every culture around the world. Making broth from grass-fed and pastured bones is how we heal not only the intestines, but also all of those digestive organs I was talking about. Bone broth has all of those amazing nutrients women spend thousands of dollars on every year: glucosamine, collagen, L-glutamine, chondroitin, calcium, magnesium, potassium, phosphorus.[23] These vitamins, minerals, and amino acids are essential for healthy digestion and metabolism. Bone broth also contains natural versions of the chemicals people take to prevent heart disease, arthritis, and bone loss, among many other maladies. If we use fish bones, we will find selenium and iodine, which are extremely beneficial for thyroid conditions. The benefits of bone broth are endless and thankfully it is becoming quite a common food. There are even several restaurants around the country that only serve bone broth. For more info check out *Nourishing Broths* written by Kaayla Daniel and Sally Fallon or *The Bone Broth Diet* by Kellyann Petrucci. These amazing reads will transform your understanding of gut health and how truly important it is for not only our nervous system, immune system, and cardio vascular system, but our metabolism as well.

Bone broth is not a joke food, it's a true superfood and currently unmeasured in its ability to heal the body. I use it in all of my client protocols. Get your gut right and you will see your life change.

The gut is also where we can begin to fight anxiety, depression, and mood disorders. If you like setting attainable goals, using food as medicine is one to strive for.

The Essential Importance Of Prebiotic And Probiotic Fibers

Once the intestines are healing from removing crap foods, drinking bone broth, and eating fermented foods, we start to understand the importance of prebiotic and probiotic fibers for healthy gut bacteria. Prebiotics are the food that probiotic bacteria eat. We usually refer to them as fiber.

Everyone is consumed with the word *fiber*, and this is what got us into such trouble to begin with. We became obsessed with a word we knew nothing about. We let the food industry run wild with a word we thought we understood, but we did not. Enter the high-fiber food products and supplements. Some people are constipated from a mineral deficiency that has nothing to do with fiber and they most likely got that deficiency from the highly processed high-fiber foods they were consuming. I know, it seems complicated, but it really comes down to focusing on the GMO and highly processed wheat and grain products that are stripping us of nutrients.

Prebiotic and probiotic fibers, coupled with fermented foods, optimal enzymatic release (the body's production of digestive enzymes: amylase, protease, lipase), and digestive function make our daily constitution optimal. So, what are they? Vegetables. People do not eat enough vegetables. Over 40 percent of our plate should be filled with vegetables.[24]

This doesn't mean that we have to be vegan or vegetarian, but it does mean that our body probably isn't getting what it needs. Variety is also very important, as all vegetables have different nutrient properties and density.

Did you know that spinach is super high in iron, protein, vitamin K, folate, copper, zinc, choline, B6, B1, B2, magnesium, and vitamin C? For lack of a better word, spinach is amazing! If you could eat your vitamins, wouldn't you?

Personally, I only spend money on supplements I know I can't get from food.

Vegetables are essential for a proper population of gut bacteria and for better digestion, metabolism, and overall system function. Different vegetables are recognized as prebiotic and probiotic fibers, they break down and feed the healthy bacteria. The body is built to eat an abundance of roughage, predominantly vegetables. We love Brussels sprouts in my house. Cruciferous vegetables, such as broccoli, cauliflower, Brussels sprouts, and kale are not only great as prebiotic fiber; they also have special enzymes that remove excessive estrogen from the digestive tract, thus helping with hormonal imbalances that cause unnecessary and toxic adipose tissue to develop.[25]

On the other hand, for some women, when discussing "bioindividuality" spinach and cruciferous vegetables can be labeled as foods inflammatory to the thyroid in those with special sensitivity to these foods. Like I have said time and time again, all bodies are different and one size will not fit all. Regardless vegetables, no matter their nutrient content or make up, are insanely important and should be seen as a primary in all meals!!

RELAXATION AND ENZYMES ARE YOUR GUT'S BEST FRIEND

Some folks out there don't do well with raw vegetables or salads and attribute that to their not being able to digest them. Well, you may not be able to at the moment, but that doesn't mean your body was built that way. Somewhere along the way you lost the proper enzymes to break these foods down. You may not relax and enjoy your meals, making it impossible for the body to properly digest your foods, especially vegetables.

Remember when I said that digestion begins in the brain and how salivary amylase is released to break down vegetable carbohydrate? Your body cannot break down vegetables unless you are in a parasympathetic state.

We need to sit, relax, breathe, and let our saliva gather so that we can dissolve the fibers we are about to eat. It is also super important to chew our food thoroughly. So many people wolf down their meals and don't savor or truly enjoy the process of eating. Mechanisms are put in place for a reason and sitting and chewing our food is primary to healthy digestion. If we are on the go, stressed out, eating quickly, and usually end up gassy and bloated from our vegetables, we might benefit from recalibrating our approach.

I know some people are going to read this and say, "I don't have time for that." Of course, you do. Truth bomb: You choose either to make or not to make the time to take care of yourself.

Women in American culture are obsessed with going a million miles a minute and often don't create healthy and mindful rituals to live by. I sit down and eat a home cooked meal six to seven nights a week, around the same time of night, always with my husband. We eat together; it's our bonding time. I make time to sit and eat my breakfast and I take the extra time to sit and eat my lunch. I sit at every meal and give myself plenty of time to relax and digest. Something to think about, if we require 40 percent of our food to be vegetables, and we have to relax in order to break them down, produce the proper enzymes for digestion, absorption, and gut bacteria production, relaxation might be the easiest answer to what some of us are dealing with in our health and wellness journey.

The Importance Of Herbs And Vitamins

When you have made the changes we have already covered, and your digestion just isn't absorbing the nutrients you need it to, or your foods are not as nutrient dense as you need them to be, it might be time to explore herbs and vitamins. Herbs have been used for thousands of years as powerful medicine.

When I began my journey into understanding my body better, of course I went to the vitamin and supplement aisle. It is an easy transition and I can be known as quite the product junkie. I was working at a local grocer as a cheese buyer at the time and the Health and Beauty buyer was one of the kindest people I worked with. She would give me samples all the time, and when I told her about different symptoms I was experiencing, she would give me a remedy. That friendship was one of my earliest encounters with a modern healer. I started taking herbs that targeted different parts of my body. I took adrenal adaptogens, such as lemon balm, holy basil, and ashwagandha, to help my stress levels. I increased my vitamin D3 intake to help increase my intake of all major nutrients. I used isolated amino acids that targeted different parts of the brain and nervous system to help me process better. I took a B complex to even out my stress levels.

I also started to experiment with glandulars, or animal organ supplements. It turned out that my body really needed them. We can't always get everything we need from food; sometimes we need a concentrated dosage of nutrients. Herbs are great for anyone who is nutrient depleted. I also got into concentrated liquid herbs called tinctures. They slowly became a part of my own remedy arsenal. I now have at least ten bottles of different tinctures for different uses. I have one called "serious relaxer," it is an instant absorber and after only four to six drops I feel really good. I only use it in extreme cases of stress, but it does the trick.

Sourcing your herbs properly is very important. You always want your herbs to be 100 percent organic and not cut, or mixed, with toxic binders. Also, making sure herbs do not contraindicate with your medications or illnesses is very important. I found out what worked for me by doing research and listening to my body. The information is at your fingertips; it just takes time to figure it all out.

I have worked with so many women over the years and have seen so many different scales and variations of what works for people and what doesn't. In the past I, have seen women respond very well to using Ashwaganda as an adrenal supplement with or without thyroid conditions. On the other hand, I have had a client who was so sensitive to it she would immediately get nauseous and vomit. The body responds so differently to all protocols, I could go on and on about what worked and what didn't for each and every man/woman I have worked with, but I think that will become a distraction to you go on your own journey.

We should all always be experts of our own bodies, because we are our only advocates. To advocate for ourselves we must be open to change, open to possibility, open to acceptance, and most importantly open to feeling as though we deserve to be happy.

CHAPTER 4
Vulnerability

Vulnerability sounds like truth and feels like courage. Truth and courage aren't always comfortable, but they're never weakness.

Brené Brown

You may feel as if you don't deserve happiness, or that your life is always going to be like this. Change is never easy. For some, the simple act of cutting their hair can be devastating, let alone changing their entire mindset and engaging in an emotional behavior like vulnerability.

We are becoming so disconnected from ourselves and our communities that we find truth and vulnerability in other people annoying. They make us uncomfortable. When we observe a person going through a difficult time, we would rather they not share that with us.

What is the point of existing if not to experience real human emotion? I know people who don't cry or avoid crying because of the fear that it will make them look weak, or that once they start, they won't be able to stop.

When Did Emotion Become Weakness?

How sad that we live in a society that promotes inhibiting our nature as a human to feel and experience emotion. The close friends in my life choose me because I love them for what they think are the ugliest parts of their life and character. I don't like to be friends with anyone unless they allow themselves to be vulnerable and express all of their "flaws" to me deeply. Life would be boring otherwise. I try to engage in fulfilling and deep relationships with people for the fact that it gives my life purpose. What I mean by that is that witnessing real human emotion is seeing true beauty. Being able to feel is the ultimate gift. Emotion connects us.

Finding our happy weight is about so many things that are connected. They are all one. If we learn how to truly express ourselves through vulnerability we become more transparent and honest, not only with others, but with ourselves. If we first accept our reality, share it, and hear it, it becomes real, and not so scary. If we keep these bits of information all locked up we create pain, we manifest disease.

One of my best girlfriends kept a secret about her health for years because she was afraid that her friends would judge her. She was afraid that if people knew, her friends would desert her. She kept the secret to herself and it ended up causing conflict in other areas of her life. It became such a fearful experience for her to imagine her secret being discovered that when she finally told me, she was emotionally devastated. Keeping something like that bottled up for so long was unbearable. She felt defeated and crippled by her inability to be vulnerable about this situation. It kept her from dating and being honest with new people. It literally controlled every decision she made. Her secret owned her.

Imagine for a second what that kind of stress does to you. Imagine what it does to your heart, your mind, and your body. Imagine how having a hidden secret could make you respond differently to every conversation, no matter how casual. Imagine how insecure or self-judging you would become. Hidden pain can cause so much stress that you lose sight of what is real. You forget to live your life. You live with pain and regret. Living with that kind of pain would never allow you to achieve complete happiness or help you to be your best self. You would never find your happy weight.

Eventually I began to push her more, encouraging her to face her fears. It took some time, but after she opened up to everyone, it was as though she had a new lease on life. She felt like herself again. She eventually started dating and she felt free. She felt like she had been let out of some kind of emotional prison. Eventually her light came back and she felt healthier than she had in years. She was in control of her life again. Vulnerability can give us the ultimate gift. But we can only gain it through truth and complete honesty about our self with others.

Being Fake Is The Ugliest Form Of Being Human

I don't believe in or encourage the act of falsifying or masking your true self. What's the point? Most "mysterious" people I know are never truly satisfied with their life and are always searching for something else. The people I feel have it the most together are the ones that are honest about their lives.

I know way too many people that keep everything to themselves and only share choice bits and pieces with people they are close to. It's so boring! How are people supposed to know how to comfort you if you hide everything? Silent sufferers and martyrs are so passé. Vulnerability is one of the main keys to finding your happy weight because if you are honest with others, you are forced to be honest with yourself.

On the other hand, honesty can get some people in a rough

situation. No one likes a victim or a chronic whiner. These are the types of people that constantly seek sympathy for an issue that is repetitive or ended ages ago. We need to be more along the lines of acting mindfully and not vulnerably, they are not mutually exclusive. To be aware of your feelings, and to express them, are two separate actions. Most victim-minded individuals are unaware of what is really happening and they get stuck in a negative loop that placates reality, but is unfortunately, fantasy. I have some family members that live in a fantasy that all of the negativity in their life just happened to them. Like they weren't a part of their lives, like they had no control.

The truth is, we all have control; we all have a choice. Yes, bad things happen, but what you do with that and how you choose to speak your story is up to you. What I mean by that is, life is what you make it. That is a theme we are going to experience through this journey.

As my mother always says, life is about choices. However, our choice only defines us until we decide to make a different one. I know that seems a little farfetched, but every second we have in this life is an opportunity to completely change ourselves. And when we make that change and stick to it, no one will even remember what came before. We'll bring up something from the past in a conversation of nostalgia and people will go, "Oh yeah, I totally forgot about that." True story!

If someone choses to repetitively remind you of something negative from the past, she is either not dealing with her own issues attached to that situation, or is so insecure that she needs to direct negative attention to you and avoid the attention on her. That's blatant projecting.

But I'm not here to give you another psychology lesson. All I will say is that this is your journey, not theirs. Don't give them the attention they are so desperately seeking, it is a complete waste of your time and energy.

Why Do You Care So Much?

Vulnerability is the act of not caring what people think. Vulnerability is about owning your emotions, feeling them physically, understanding them visually, and sharing them audibly. Understanding your feelings visually is the act of picturing the scenario. For example, I remember the moment I said goodbye to my grandmother for the last time, she had just had a stroke. She was so blissfully unaware of the tragedy that was unfolding around her. When I told her I loved her and that I was going to miss her she smiled and replied "I love you", so beautifully, unknowingly about to leave the physical world she knew.

Visualizing this moment, forever frozen in my mind, allows me to feel something amazing and life changing. As I sit here writing this, tears are streaming down my face. I am reliving the experience all over again. A moment like this is not to be hidden or feel shamed over. This was a real moment in my life that I never want to forget or feel numb towards.

Vulnerability is one of the many wonderful things we are capable of. It is the way in which we express our self and work through emotion. In *Women's Bodies Women's Wisdom,* Christiane Northrup, M.D., one of the most acclaimed and successful obstetrician-gynecologists in the country, discusses the process of unexpressed emotional trauma manifesting into disease. She says that we can actually create physical disease if we do not have resolution from emotional trauma.[1] The very lack of expressing our feelings physically or verbally can kill us. If we're afraid of being vulnerable and expressing our self, it is time to work through the fear for the sake of saving our life.

Expressing emotion through the act of vulnerability without shame or guilt can be so freeing that it can truly release us from a diseased state.

Asking For Help Is Not Weakness

Vulnerability is also about being able, and knowing when,

to ask for help. There is nothing wrong with asking for help if you truly need it. This is something I still struggle with on a daily basis, but have gotten increasingly better at over the years. My husband says it's because of the chip I have on my shoulder. Others say it is because of my stubborn nature. I like to think of it as strength. But strengths can become weaknesses if we do not accept the power of vulnerability.

We get so caught up in our own agendas that we forget that people like to be helpful, and love to be a part of our process. Why else do we think they are a part of our life? They want to be near us, support us, love us, whether or not we believe that to be true.

I tend to be a secretly competitive person and don't typically ask for help. I usually want to do everything on my own. The need to be alone is the ugly side of competition; when we are alone we become paranoid, jealous, and egotistical. Asking for help humbles us and makes us a part of a team. Collaboration is what makes an idea or a situation worthwhile, because we have someone to share it with.

No one likes a lack of humility; it makes us look cold and callused. It sets a bad energy around us. It's like the Ronda Rousey vs. Holly Holm fight. Instead of embracing Holm as her equal and touching gloves, Rousey saw her not as an equal fighter working toward the same goal, instead she saw her as an unworthy opponent. Her ego got the best of her and she lost focus, very shortly after the fight began, she lost. I get that not touching gloves was an intimidation tactic, but it shows poor sportsmanship and can be a mental game changer. It obviously gave Holm the advantage and in turn Rousey lost a bit of credibility. The previously undefeated female bantamweight champion of the world was handed a strong slice of humble pie.

Humility is another part of vulnerability, because to be truly humble is to express a side of us that may never be seen.

Letting your guard down and living in equality in that which you fear most is to be truly vulnerable. This is not weakness! If you feel tension with another person, but refuse to hear their story or you refuse to tell yours, this is pride. Pride is weakness. The strength of being secure in one's self comes from the act of being vulnerable. Vulnerability seen as weakness is actually arrogance. To feel entitled and elitist is unskillful and unhelpful. No one person on this planet is better than the next.

Don't Be Afraid

Here is a great example of what vulnerability looks like in a social context: Imagine you are at a party with friends and strangers. You have some internal dialogue and fears or anxieties about what is going on around you. Maybe you're concerned about what other people are thinking about the food you are eating. You start making justifications, or get overwhelming anxiety about the entire situation. If you are stressed about how other people view your food choices, then you are giving those people way too much power and control over your emotions.

I know that meeting new people, or going to a new place, or being around people and food at the same time can generate a lot of fear. But why should it? Because you are afraid to draw attention to yourself! You don't want to get asked any questions about your food, healthy or not. You don't want people to know how much you really eat, so you put tiny bits on your plate. Or you overload your plate and think everyone is judging you, so you are quiet, get an attitude, or get embarrassed. There are so many unnecessary emotions involved with food in social situations. I have experienced this first hand and have helped people with this issue. I frankly don't care what people think about me when I am eating the food I want, when I want to eat it. Do you want to know why? Because it's none of their business! They don't really know me. They are not aware of my struggles with food sensitivities or my battles with emotional attachment to foods.

The bottom line is, no one has the right to judge you in anything you do, especially the food you eat. Don't be stressed about drawing attention to yourself, or being a burden on others. Humans are naturally curious know-it-alls. If you are trying something new, they will ask you what it is, why you're doing it, how you heard about it, and then tell you why it does or doesn't work. Are they professional health care providers? Of course not. But everyone thinks that because they read this one Facebook post that was shared by so and so, or follow this one blogger, they have a doctorate in health and wellness.

Try to not take these situations too seriously and always be looking out for number one, you! The less you engage in the negativity that surrounds these situations, the better and more comfortable you will feel.

You should never feel like a burden to those around you. If someone truly cares for you, they will always try their best to make you happy. At the end of the day, the only person that knows what is right for you is you. I urge you to stand tall, feel confident that you are amazing, be emotional, be vulnerable, and be you!

12 Actions To Unlock Your Vulnerability

What are my keys to unlocking your vulnerability? I believe that action is the key. We don't experience vulnerability by just thinking about it. Here is a great action list to get you started. These actions are to help overcome the fears that are keeping you from living your true life. Please be mindful and cautious.

- *Dance naked in the mirror without judging yourself.* Have you ever looked in the mirror and not thought something negative about yourself? Have you ever just looked and said, "I look amazing, I am so beautiful!" If not, then I encourage you to start by being silly. Allow yourself time to dance in front of the mirror naked with music that makes you feel the happiest. Do not even for a second think anything negative, and don't stop unless you have to!

- *Be completely positive and mindful for a whole day. Do* you realize that you are stressing your life away? I am so tired of hearing how busy people are; it's so negative. If you're actually booked every second of the day, then maybe you are busy, but when people ask you how you are, don't respond with "busy." Try being more positive and talk about all of the things that you are happy about or proud of. This makes you vulnerable because when we stop being fake, real emotion comes out.

- *Wear an outfit that is completely unlike you.* We often define ourselves by the clothes we wear. Sometimes we play it too safe, and sometimes we overdo it in order to take the attention off of the real us. Spend a few days dawning a new style in public, either wearing no makeup if you usually wear it, or wearing something sassy and eclectic if you tend to keep it simple.

- *Be Comfortable telling someone NO by simultaneously saying YES.* Say yes to life and doing the things that make you uncomfortable, while saying no to those that suck the life out of you. To be vibrant and fully existing in this world, we need to live the life we want and be in complete control of our decisions.

- *Fall in love with yourself.* We can only truly begin to make positive shifts in our lives and be completely vulnerable if we are in love with who it is we are. You are an amazing person despite what you may think of yourself. Be in love with everything you do. If you don't like what you are doing, change it, until you are truly happy. You'll get one step closer to your happy weight every time you fall in love with yourself.

- *Talk to someone that you have been silently judging.* Everyone is walking through life with fear, and everyone's fears are different. Fears make us judge people for various reasons. Talking to someone you do not know using a positive tone can ignite something positive in them. If it doesn't, you can continue to be a positive force. But I think you will be surprised by their reaction. Not all situations turn out how you envision them and the aftermath can create change in you and others involved.

- *Ask for help.* We carry the weight of the world on our shoulder and we don't often ask for help. Asking for help can be as little as letting the bag clerk carry out your groceries at the market or allowing your friend to buy you coffee for a change.

- *Do something that far exceeds your comfort zone.* Apply for that job you never thought you would get, but really want. If they say no, keep trying until you get it. Get that tattoo you've been wanting, or color your hair the way you have always dreamed. Don't let others dictate what you do with your body.

- *Take that trip you have always wanted to take even if no one wants to go with you.* Do you want to look back on your life and have regrets? Stop justifying your complacency; if you are thinking about something, it is a desire. DO IT! STOP WASTING TIME!

- *Cry in front of a complete stranger.* When was the last time you cried in front of another person that wasn't your significant other or family member? Yesterday? Last month? Last year? Never? If it's been a while, reflect on why that is. Why do you find it difficult to let others into your life, why is it so hard to cry in front of someone else? Do you feel guilt, are you ashamed, does it make you feel too exposed? Now think back to the last time you did cry in front of someone else. What happened? Was it traumatizing, were they mean to you, or did they shut you down? Sit with that. Dig deep. Give yourself the permission to cry. And NEVER apologize for crying.

- *Do a new activity alone, or with people you don't know.*

Challenging our comfort zones forces us to step outside of our day to day. We feel naked without our creature comforts. If we go somewhere without our significant other or friends, we are thrown into uncharted territory. This action makes us ask questions, engage in conversation, be a part of something that terrifies us, but can have beautiful results.

- *Do something in front of people that you are terrified of doing.* Share something that ignites your emotions at work, school, or in front of peers. Poetry, public speaking, a story from your life, or a chapter from your favorite book. The options are endless. The point is to overcome the flood of being overwhelmed in front of others and realizing that the fear is far worse than the action.

- *Invite friends over and teach them an activity you excel at.* We are completely raw and exposed when we have to represent a part of ourselves. Whether it is a creative project or a wellness exercise, the "what" doesn't matter. The "who" is the most important thing. That who is you. You will be the educator in this situation, show that you love yourself and be proud of what you do.

These are called "actions" because that is exactly what we do to experience our vulnerability, we act on it, we take action to live it. When we fully experience our vulnerability with our whole body and create an almost muscle memory of it, it in time becomes easier, we become more comfortable in our own skin. Take action, be vulnerable, be you!

CHAPTER 5
Loving Yourself By Releasing Shame And Guilt

You have been criticizing yourself for years, and it hasn't worked. Try approving of yourself and see what happens.

Louise L. Hay

A specific memory comes to mind when I think of how detrimental weight loss programs can be on a person's self-esteem. I think back to a time when I had to measure the whole body of every client. This was generally the very first appointment people would have before beginning their program. They were forced to get on a scale, have measurements done, and have their picture taken. This was explained to the client as a positive way to track progress. I now understand that this was an oppressive tactic to generate revenue. The more result we had as leverage, the more product we could sell.

I remember one new client in particular that not only became flushed during the process, but began to sweat. It didn't occur to me until much later that this woman was feeling so much emotion and stress that she began to perspire. I can only imagine how devastating an experience this must have been for her. Remember me speaking earlier about working in the ketogenic weight loss clinic and how there were employee weight requirements and dress codes as well? Not only was I a five-foot-six blond, weighing 120 pounds with a mandated body fat percentage below 27 percent, but I was also had to dress in my finest clothes. How incredibly uncomfortable and intimidating it must have been to come to a weight-loss clinic and go through this process with me. I tried to be kind, but I was a walking poster child for creating potential eating disorders.

I don't regret the life experience and education I gained on this job, but I do regret any negative feelings that may have been generated on my watch. The idea that I may be forever seared into a woman's memory regarding her self-image in a negative way makes me nauseous.

I can't speak for everyone when I say that measurements of the size of our thighs and our biceps and our stomachs, and the numbers on the scale, rule our entire lives, but I bet many of us do let them. Our age, the number on our scale, pant sizes, body measurements. It's always an ongoing competition we have created with our self and others. Some of us will tear our appearance apart and never truly appreciate the beauty that already exists. Some of us think that we have been unhappy with our body for as long as we can remember and believe it will never be perfect.

When you look back in the past, to different times in your life, when thinking about your body, is the only thing you remember the numbers? Do you remember how much you weighed on prom night, or your wedding day?

Thinking of this gives me a vivid flash of that scene from *Mean Girls*. Societies ideal of "perfectly beautiful" young women stare into the mirror and cut themselves down, together. It's disgusting. We all have differences, but why do we have to hate them so much? Why do we have to be run by a number? What is wrong with basing our health and happiness on the way we feel? Every time I ask a new client what they are expecting to achieve, they almost always say a pant size or a weight on the scale. It's hard for me to encourage this, but they are determined that this is their motivation. I also feel very uncomfortable congratulating someone on their weight loss. It is an achievement, if you have decided to focus more on your health, but is it healthy to always be given gratification after losing weight? Doesn't that type of behavior perpetuate the negative idea that we needed to change in the first place and that we are only worthy if we lose weight? Is seeking gratification from others a part of the problem as well? Can't we just be happy with our own accomplishments without looking for approval?

If you are constantly focused on being something that may not be sustainable, is that a healthy state of mind? Will you ever feel whole?

I think the overall misfortune of all of this is that we are still focusing on the past and not living in the present. Most women trying to lose weight are so focused on a number that they forget to do the work that really needs to be done: the healing.

If you weren't happy before, when you were whatever number you equate to happiness, what makes you think you will be happy and feel fulfilled this time around?

If you didn't love yourself then, what makes you think you will magically start loving yourself now?

It's time to dig deep and make peace with yourself, and make peace with whatever brought you here to this moment. It's time you quit basing your happiness on a number. Allow your heart to heal. Make the changes necessary to love yourself and the life you lead. It's time to throw away the scale; it doesn't determine your worth. Burn the jeans that you use for motivation. Toss out the measuring tapes, and calipers. Allow yourself to be free of any number that dictates how you feel about yourself.

What makes all of these people, that I see on every health tips bookshelf, experts? What happened to the good old days of eating nutrient-dense whole foods made from scratch, while being naturally active? It's time to stop dieting, and to start loving ourselves. This entire society has completely changed from what used to be so simple, and is now, so complicated. We started to see the negative effects of our changing culture in the 1950s when we started slinging diet pills laced with methamphetamines and telling women that they were fat and not good enough. Hollywood blew up and television was born. The media destroyed any idea of normalcy we had when it came to image. And every woman from then on was told daily, on every outlet, that they were not enough.

Who told you that you needed to look a certain way and be a certain size? Do you remember the first time you thought you weren't good enough, or that someone thought you weren't pretty enough, or thin enough? Did they have it all together? Does the person (or people) making you feel this way right now have it all? Probably not. Absolutely not.

Sometimes we use negative language about ourselves to get motivated and we don't realize that when we reach our goal, that negative, internal dialogue still exists. If we don't work on the emotional, the physical will never be enough. We can never achieve our happy weight if we don't first focus within.

We get so concerned with what others have because, somehow, we think their life is better than ours, or perfect, or that they know better than we do. It is completely false. How is their life better than ours? Because they look so awesome on social media? Because when we see them out on the town, or in their perfect Christmas card, they seem so happy? Social media is easy to falsify. Everyone posts the picture of themselves out on the town. No one posts the picture of them crying in a corner.

I meet fake people all the time, and I see them as just that: fake. I would never aspire to be like someone that doesn't appear to have flaws, because it isn't real. I have a few friends that only tell people what they need to hear so that everyone will think they are impervious to life's negatives. They absolutely are not. They are no more superior in their existence than I am or you are. I honestly believe that the reason people are followed by others and become leaders is because most people don't think they are capable of making changes themselves. We are full of an idea that somehow another person will give us salvation, as if we need to be saved from something. If we do need to be saved from something and we make it out, the only credit that should ever be given is to us. We are the one that went to that meeting, or read that book, we are the one that ran that marathon, or ended a toxic relationship. We can and should thank people for support, our friends and loved ones for encouraging us, but if we don't start to believe that we are the leader of our own lives, we will never be truly present. We will always rely on others to be the drivers of our destiny.

I'm sure you have heard the word *mindfulness* being thrown around, but maybe haven't understood the meaning entirely. Mindfulness is the art of being present. Mindfulness teaches us the truth about our lives and our self. To be truly mindful puts us in a position where we can be objective about our lives and see things clearly. For example, did you know that hunger can be mistaken for thirst? Most of us don't know we are dehydrated until it's too late.

This is just one of the many examples of stepping outside of your busy mind and tapping into our innate intelligence. Asking questions like, Am I really hungry or am I thirsty? Am I really angry, or am I just hungry? Does she really have it all, or are we the same, and does she envy me too?

Mindfulness is a challenge for all of us in many different areas, but it is also the key to digging deep inside of our mind and asking the difficult questions. Am I truly happy? Why do I feel this way? If we don't engage in the act of mindful living every so often, we do not pose these questions and move through the problem. Holding diplomatic conversation is something that occurs in my household daily, we take a very Socratic approach: Listen, ask, answer positively.

If we answer definitively, we close ourselves off room for other options. Most of the time our definitive answers come from a learned idea. Learned ideas and behaviors can be hard to change if we are not willing to step outside of the box and see what is waiting for us on the other side. We must be ready for any amount of change, because if we are not ready or fully committed to the cause, we will revert back to old habits. These learned ideas and behaviors are things someone has said or done that anchor inside of us and makes us believe that this is the only truth. But the only truth is whatever we want it to be.

The one truth is that there are no rules to this life. You can make it any way you want and live any life you want.

Some women deal with the demons of their family's past. For example, maybe one time your mother or father said something horrible to you, like "You're ugly," "You'll never be able to do that," "You're too fat for that," or "You'll never look like that." This is shameful and hurtful, and these words should never be said to anyone. I have heard these statements before and thought, *What a horrible thing it would be to hear this. Why would anyone ever speak to another person like this? How damaged can one person be to deliberately cut another person down like this?*

Then I have asked myself, *What happened to the person saying this, that they felt the need to be so cruel?* When I ask this type of question I begin to have compassion for this person, because someone before her most likely said the same thing to her. Negativity is a perpetual notion that doesn't divert unless we change the emotion or behavior. My parents hate that I have tattoos, for example, but at the end of the day, I am who I want to be and if they want to be in my life, they have to deal with it. Luckily, they do, and through my constant motion of challenging their ideas of truth, they have become more open and accepting people. People can change, they do all the time. If they don't change, it's because they don't want to.

First and foremost, turn the focus on yourself. It's time for you to think about yourself and the things you want and need out of this life. Where do you start? It's all candy and gum drops reading about how you got to where you are today, but how do you make a change from here?

Let's start with the easiest part, because we all know how to do this. Let's make a list. Below is an example of a possibilities list, the possibilities of what you want and what you need. Write one separately on a piece of paper. When you are done fold it up and leave it in the book I really want you look back later in this process and see where you began. This is going to be a very different kind of list than some you may have made in the past, because we are going to use the steps of vulnerability we learned in the last chapter. This possibilities list is a serious reflection of what plagues us and what attainable goals we would like to move toward.

I have written some examples on the list below to give you a bit of guidance into what you are trying to accomplish here.

Take some time to truly write out fears and positive possibilities so that you can look back and reflect on your transformation.

When we fully live in our truth and accept the changes we want and need so desperately to make, then we can move forward into our health and wellness journey, we can start to own the decisions we make.

My Fears of Change and
the Positive Possibilities of the Outcome

Fears	Possibilities
Ex: Say **NO** to something	When you say NO you are instantly free from that obligation! Don't be ashamed or feel guilty to live the life YOU want!
*Say NO to something you don't want to do like an activity you clearly don't like but typically agree to out of obligation	
Ex: Say **YES** to something	If you say YES You are Empowered to make decisions for yourself and are free of the control we can feel of others decisions
*This can make us feel as though we are monopolizing the situation or that no one will want to be a part of whatever it is we want to do	

CHAPTER 6
Breaking Up Is Hard To Do

Two words. Three vowels. Four consonants. Seven letters. It can either cut you open to the core and leave you in ungodly pain or it can free your soul and lift a tremendous weight off your shoulders. The phrase is: It's over.

Maggi Richard

If inflammation is the root cause of disease, the answer should be simple, right? Remove the foods causing inflammation. Unfortunately, it's not that simple. These food choices are deeply rooted and emotionally driven. If we were a society that ate to live and didn't live to eat, we wouldn't be having this discussion.

So what is inflammation? Inflammation is a localized protective response elicited by injury or destruction of tissues, which serves to destroy, dilute, or wall off both the injurious agent and the injured tissue.[1] It can alter blood pH, causing things like arthritis, or alter the gut flora, causing intestinal disorders like

Crohn's disease or irritable bowel syndrome (IBS). Inflammation can alter how the brain reacts in the cases of multiple sclerosis or Lyme disease. Inflammation can directly affect the endocrine system causing estrogen dominance, adrenal fatigue, or thyroid disorder.[2]

How do we prevent it? By altering our eating habits and lifestyle choices. Seems simple, yet is so difficult for most, mainly because we don't know where to start, and we are addicted to the food America feeds us.

Let Food Be Your Medicine

If used correctly, food can heal our deeper issues. We know that breaking up is hard to do. We also know that it is often absolutely necessary. The right foods can fix metabolic dysfunction and reverse most things that inhibit us from being healthy. I know so many women that hide behind their diseases like hypothyroidism and PCOS, blame all of their metabolic issues on the disease, and give up. That is not the correct way to approach health, as becoming a victim of our disease will leave us empty and sick.

I knew a girl once who came to me when I worked in weight loss and said that because of her PCOS, it was impossible to lose weight, though she continued to drink wine and eat fried foods every day. Which one do you think caused her issues? On the other hand, I helped to guide one woman with both PCOS and Hashimoto's disease in giving up her addiction to sugar and gluten. Through a clean eating plan, a relaxation practice, loving herself, and attending some yoga classes, she was able to achieve health goals she hadn't seen in years. After all, it's not about the number we see on that scale, it's about our energy, our self-worth, and our overall health. However, we can't reach any goals if we are not ready to make a change in the foods we eat.

The modern definition of using food as medicine is as follows: Eat to heal your body, eat to balance hormones, eat to increase positive neurochemicals, eat to sleep better, eat to reduce stress (not create more), eat to reduce inflammation, eat to reverse your disease and not continue to suffer from it. All of the ways to achieve using food as medicine are here in this book. Listen, research, and find your path to living a healthier and fuller life.

Which Food Is More Important Than Your Health?

Which food is so important that you can't give it up? None, not a single one! It's not the food that makes you hesitate; it is the loss of whatever emotional tie you have to that food. You may not even realize that you are emotionally reacting, or that there will be a feeling of significant loss when you stop eating that food.

The truth is that we eat three or more times a day, 365 days a year. We need to eat to survive, and as emotional beings, naturally we become emotionally attached to our food. We use food too as a coping mechanism at so many times throughout our lives. We eat in celebration of life at birthday parties and weddings and anniversaries. We eat when we see a friend or go for a work meeting. We feed a friend or loved one when they have lost someone and are experiencing grief. We have absolutely no way to differentiate the many emotions we experience when eating. One special meal can represent an entire relationship.

Remember my grandmother, my Nonie? She was the light of my life, and to this day my memories of her are some of my absolute favorite. She taught me to love cooking and baking, she taught me how to make blackberry jam, and how to harvest and steam clams.

My grandparents meant everything to me. They were and will always be two of the most significant people that contributed to my character.

My favorite meal of all time is Chicken Divan, because that's what my Nonie made every time she saw me. It brings tears to my eyes as I write this because of the emotion that exists around this memory. These emotions are attached to every fiber of my being. This food will forever be a part of my story, my history.

This is the same for any person that has a story, good, bad, or indifferent. Food makes us feel, because it is how we express ourselves and how we nourish our bodies. I cook for the people dearest to me, according to their dietary needs because it is one way I share my love with them.

Now think about the memories you have and what they mean to you. You can begin to understand why we are all addicted to food. Food is something that makes us feel alive and in control. Just sit with that for a moment and absorb what I am trying to tell you. Food is what we need to survive, but what foods we choose determines whether we simply survive, or fully thrive.

It is inevitable that if you decide to break up with a certain food after reading this book, you will experience a form of loss, significant or not. And you will express emotion from this separation. It may sound trivial to some, but honor every emotion you experience through this process, and give yourself permission to grieve. Give yourself permission to grieve the loss of this food that once gave you joy, but has now become harmful to your health. I'm not saying you have to give up your creature comforts, just shift them a little, I still eat bread, now it's just gluten free bread and I'm not horribly sick after every meal.

This transition is also an opportunity to think about where this emotion stems from. Why are you grieving the loss of a particular food? Why is it so hard for you to make this change? It is because you are still worried about what others think?

Honestly though, why do you care so much about what others think? Did you know that almost every person you meet will think that you are judging them too? No one cares about what you are eating, what you are wearing, or what you said. If they do, then they are mirroring their own insecurity. Unless someone said something rude directly to you, or hurt your feelings in some way, they are most likely a nice person and are just as afraid as you are. We all can learn a little from giving each other some credit. If we judge them less, they will judge us less. Are you judging them because they show you something about yourself that you don't like?

I know plenty of people that think someone is overweight despite being almost exactly the same size as that person. They in turn, think that person is gross and are completely unaware that they are unhappy with themselves. This is a mirror of their own self-hatred. Don't project your insecurities and fears onto others. Rather, be a positive force, love yourself, and love others in the process.

Express your feelings so others know how to help and be of service to you, and comfort you when you need it. No one knows how you feel until you express your feelings. Fear is removed when you are truly vulnerable and verbally express your deepest fears.

Let's go back to the party scenario from the chapter on vulnerability. This goes out particularly to the people who continue to eat processed junk food. You know that the processed food you're eating on occasion, or all the time, is bad for you but you keep eating it. You keep eating it not because you like it but because you think you're not supposed to have it and therefore it's a treat. You can continue to eat this food if you want to, because it's your life and I'm not telling you what you should or shouldn't do. This is your life and your choice. However, when did processed foods that contribute to disease become a treat? That sounds like a trick to me. Maybe you feel like you are stuck in a vicious cycle of judgment and you binge eat foods that you know you don't really want to eat. But why?

We binge because of the fear of losing the choice. It's that simple. When choice is taken away from anyone they will rebel. We might say "I refuse to give up gluten!" or "I like fast food," or "It's too hard," even though it is clearly contributing to our health issues. What is really happening here? The process is emotional for us. There are hundreds of gluten-, dairy-, grain-, nut-, egg-, and nightshade-free recipes that will rock our world. There are healthy fast food options, and many of the well-trained holistic professionals ready to be our support system, but we still hesitate. What emotions that you have connected to your food are you still holding on to? Why are you "living to eat" and not "eating to live"?

FEAR INHIBITS CHANGE

We are afraid; it is all fear related. We are afraid to change, afraid of what others will think, afraid that our perfectly calculated life will change, afraid that everything we knew to be right is wrong, and afraid that we really do have problems with food. But the only person who cares about this is us! The only thing the people in our life care about is our health, because they want to keep us around. Or maybe we are their only friend willing to make a change and they are afraid to be left out. How sad is that? Should our friends be encouraging each other to live with disease rather than defeating it? That sounds toxic to me.

So if you're ready to change and take your health seriously, here is my six-step guide to move you forward and help you break up with harmful foods:

1. You must be mentally prepared to take a leap of faith and change everything you know to be true about the foods you are eating. If you are not ready to break up with the foods that are causing you pain and inhibiting you from finding your happy weight, then come back later when you have realized that you do have control over your choices and are truly ready.

2. Every bite, lick, or taste affects you no matter what you convince yourself to be true. Remember you are going to stop lying to yourself. "Treats" and "cheats" are emotional escapes from the reality you are refusing to deal with.

3. If you make a choice that isn't according to plan, don't feel guilty; instead try harder to understand why you made that choice, what you were feeling, and what your experience was-having made that choice. These moments exist to educate you on how to make different choices that affect your life positively. If you bring guilt into your life, you are not fully embracing yourself as a strong, confident woman.

4. Stop being picky. Step outside of your comfort zone and try something new! Trust me, foods that are new and foreign to you, that you are not allergic to, won't kill you.

5. Take control of conversations with people involving your food choices. Beware of feeders! A feeder is a person that forces food or conversations about your food choices on you every time you see them. Speak up, make your needs known, and say no. Your health is more important than the risk of being rude.

6. Remember to eat something pleasurable at least once a day. Food is a gift that nourishes us, enjoy it. Find foods that bring you pleasure and that don't bring you harm. There are many allergen-free foods that can bring your palate pleasure.

This six-step plan will help you realize that you have the power to do anything you set your mind to. If you think you are incapable of change, or that you are not strong enough, think again! You are absolutely capable of making any changes you have ever wanted to make in your life. Breaking up with food is half the battle; the rest is living in your new truth.

If that means you lose a few friends in the process, or move to a new town, so be it. Give yourself permission to be exactly who you want to be. Make no apologies, and make no excuses. Start to live the life that makes you happy, healthy, and balanced. When you are on your deathbed, you do not want to look back with regret.

If it is not a food that you need to break up with, it may be a disease, or the negativity you are feeding yourself. I have a friend that I admire quite a lot. She is a beautiful creature that sees the world in a light that most people don't. She has Hashimoto's, and although she used to engulf herself in living an autoimmune lifestyle, and spent hours on all of the blogs and forums, she woke up one day and decided to break up with her disease, to not let it define her. She moved to a whole new country to find freedom from the life she had been living, and to gain perspective. She did not avoid experiencing all of the emotion that came with so much change, but she felt renewed rather than overwhelmed. The idea that her disease did not define her gave her an entirely new lease on life. She felt energized because her obsession with being perfect disappeared and she focused on her image of herself, not the image others had of her. It made her feel whole again.

Searching for community and belonging to new tribes should always feel good and make us happy. The second that it doesn't, it is time to make a change and break free, shed our former self, and experience a rebirth. No matter what we believe in, the one thing we cannot deny as humans is that we are ever growing, ever changing, and like the natural world we live in, we need to cleanse ourselves and reshape our lives. If we are being held back for whatever reason, break free! Don't give into stagnation! Be confident!

Tips And Tricks For Success

Going gluten-free was very hard for me, emotionally, but I overcame it. I endured the challenges of change. There were times when all I wanted was to eat every baked good in the display case that I walked by. I found some advice helped more than others, and so I offer to you a short list of mantras for when the challenge seems too much.

- *Accept your reality to be true.* Stop allowing tiny excuses to be a part of your existence. Start slowly, but accept the truth. Where you are now is not where you want to be.

- *Love yourself completely.* All of the flaws you have are a part of what makes you human and beautiful. Accept this to be true. You are priceless. You can do anything.

- *Set tangible and attainable goals for yourself.* Big or small, set them for every step of the way. If you make goals that are out of your reach, you are less likely to follow through. Example: Plan to walk once a week until you get a groove and want to do it more, as opposed to saying you are going to run every day. Starting, not doing, is the hardest part.

- *Stop apologizing for everything!* Why do you need to say sorry when you have done nothing wrong? Only apologize if you have truly done wrong, otherwise remove sorry from your daily vocabulary. It is a weakness that you no longer have time for. Apologizing for everything doesn't make you humble, it makes you easy to take advantage of.

- *Remove yourself from negative situations.* The same goes for people that keep you from moving forward. Only do something if you feel happy and accomplished afterward. If you feel guilty, forced, or uncomfortable, it might not be the right fit.

- *Try everything more than once.* Sometimes negative feelings can be nerves in a new environment.

- *Set yourself free and never look back, unless it is to reflect.* Changing your path to wellness doesn't separate you from who you truly are. It just changes your views on food, not your views on life.

CHAPTER 7
True Confidence: The Act Of Giving Yourself Permission

Shoot for the moon. Even if you miss you'll land among the stars.

Norman Vincent Peale

What does it even mean to give yourself permission? The first time I heard it, it didn't make sense. Give myself permission to do what exactly? The answer is: permission to live the life you want. If you want to eat dessert, eat it. Don't beat yourself up or hate yourself because of a food choice you made. Be confident in your decisions. Be the person you want to be, express any and all emotions whenever you feel like it. Give yourself permission to experience all this life has to offer. Who is watching you anyway? Why are you nervous or looking over your shoulder? Who is policing you? Aren't you a grown woman, capable of making her own decisions?

Women often forget to give themselves permission to be

free. We are so concerned with what others think that we drive ourselves crazy with responsibility and accusation. We think somehow, somewhere, we were given this duty to take care of everyone and everything that comes into our lives. But why? Why are we so burdened with having to make sure everything in our path is so perfect? Humans are fallible. It is a psychological fact. We are not perfect.

Our Competitive Nature

We are, however, overly competitive, whether we admit it or not. Competition is not confidence. Competition can sometimes create a very healthy drive in individuals, while in others it may contribute to their downfall. Competition often breeds insecurity. At some point, we were convinced that we weren't capable of something. The fear of failure that was created by that air of competition influences us for a lifetime. Somehow looks, education, and monetary value have become our global markers of self-worth. Some of us look to magazines, Pinterest, or our community for an image. We create stories in our head that so-and-so has it all figured out and we need to be exactly like them. We compare our body to theirs, we look at what they are ordering for lunch, and we stalk their Instagram to see what perfect photo they took that day. We ultimately feel defeated by this competition and comparison. We forget that public personas are made up. They are fabricated for our viewing pleasure. A nice camera and good positioning can make anyone look "perfect." It is all really nonsense, though. Not one single person on this planet eats perfectly 100 percent of the time. Every body is so incredibly different, and fitness and health shouldn't be made to look perfect and easy. They are not, they take work, dedication, and bravery.

As a society though, we create these systems. Some of us are obsessed with them. I know so many people that have to have everything perfect, so they feel that they are keeping up with the Joneses.

For me, this couldn't be further from my truth. I understand that, yes, I need to make money in order to live in today's world, but I don't need to make millions or be friends with people who do. I don't need to go to a special religious center or church to "be seen." I don't need to have a higher education from an Ivy League school to fit in with an elitist crowd. I don't need to belong to a country club or social group in order to be a part of something.

We are a community-driven, label-driven, and status-driven species. But at what cost? Are we actually happy if we have all of these things? No, of course not. I know so many unhappy rich people, so many unhappy "good-looking" people, so many unhappy leaders and educators. The truth is, the only reason so many people think they can't do things is because they see someone else achieve something that seems impossible, and think somehow that that other person is blissfully happy. That assumption couldn't be further from the truth. Confidence doesn't come from becoming someone else, or from an idea others have of you.

CONFIDENCE WILL HELP YOU FULFILL YOUR DESTINY

Confidence is about fulfilling your destiny and dreams of becoming the person you would be proud to be. It means no longer hiding behind someone else's idea of you, or some false persona that doesn't feel right to you. If you like being material-istic, vapid, shallow, and elitist, by all means, pursue that dream. I'll be over here, content with the fact that I am living my life and fulfilling the destiny that I set in motion long ago. Confidence is found inside of you. Confidence is about forgetting horrible things you or another has said about you, and moving into a perpetually positive mindset. Confidence is found in the deepest part of yourself, the darkest part, the saddest part, the hardest part, the most exhilarating and exciting part. You find confidence in saying NO to others' wills and wishes. You will regret letting someone else be the driver of your life.

RELIVING MY ROAD TO CONFIDENCE

As a young girl, I was very intimidated by life. The only solace I found from social insecurities was my alone time. I played with my dolls and fantasized about a life outside the one I had, because like I said earlier, I was always the new girl. Kids are mean, awkward, and territorial, regurgitating whatever ugliness their parents have spoon fed them. At school my teachers were my only saving grace. They saw things in me that I couldn't see, and fought for me every step of the way. I was never in a city long enough to get a comfortable routine. For some, this can be devastating. For me, the outcome was glorious.

As each year passed, I found routine in language, music, outdoor sports, and those summers with my grandparents. The summers were my ultimate break from the reality I knew, and taught me to appreciate the things that came before my time. At twelve years old, I fell madly in love with classic films, vinyl 45s, and blackberry picking. Those summers gave my inconsistent life a strong foundation. I was the weird girl in high school that liked classical jazz, folk, blues, and foreign language. I loved gothic art and religious history. I was obsessed with French cheese and liver pâté. My Orange County High School girlfriends still make jokes about my awkwardness today. This isn't my soap box moment, I just want you to know that through all of this insecurity, adversity, and change, I always looked at the positive. Was I emotional and moody sometimes? Of course, I'm human. But at the end of the day I said, "Yes" to most of the opportunities I was presented.

Often our insecurities can overwhelm us so much that we say no to life, close ourselves off, and hide behind excuses as to why we can't do something. At one point in my life, I was so insecure that my anxiety kept me from ordering pizza over the phone. I felt uncomfortable taking a leading role in any activity. One day I decided to just push myself into any and everything I could- and began saying YES to life.

I wanted to say yes to life so much, that I made that life altering choice at 15 and I left for Norway.

I'm not sure if you got the gist before, but Norway is an amazing country of community, history, and equality. Responsibility and age structures are unlike anything I have ever seen. This journey into another world quickly became a part of my soul and taught me to truly live my life outside of the box I grew up in. By the end of my year there, like I said before, I was a different person, I went from a girl to a woman. I could be nude with no shame, I could enjoy conversation about the social structures I believed in, and I was no longer an outsider in my community because I had found a new one. The people I experienced gave me more friendship and acceptance than I have ever experienced from a community up to that point. They pushed me beyond my limitations and believed in me until I believed in myself. If you can, try to imagine going to a place that embodies the complete opposite of what you have been taught about society, relationships, acceptance, and possibility.

I was supported in the idea that every woman is beautiful and that body positivity does exist. That aging naturally is beautiful, and being natural is beautiful. I will never forget the love and adoration I received from the friends I made and still have today.

Next move was to college at seventeen. It was a rollercoaster of learning and disaster. For the first time, I had a boyfriend longer than a few months and had roommates as well. I look back and sometimes regret that I didn't go to a school that was more in line with my personality. But, regrets give the past too much credit. Every opportunity and experience in this life is a chance to learn something. I met some very wonderful people along that journey. I was able to have many adventurous sexual experiences that helped me to become more comfortable and confident with what kind of pleasure I like. Sex is huge, and Americans are too prudish. So many divorces come from people being unsatisfied at a basic level. If you don't know how to be pleased, you will resent your partner.

I do not share my story to make you feel as though you haven't done enough, or experienced enough. I only want to show you an example of the amazing things that can come from saying yes! That's all, nothing more. This is a story about how saying yes can grow confidence.

At twenty-two, I moved to China and was living a crazy life. This was 2006-2007, and the yuan-to-dollar conversion rate was seven to one. Things were super cheap and I had the most amazingly unforgettable year. My Beijing crew and I called ourselves the Inner Circle. This is our ten-year anniversary and we are now like family. It was a beautiful unforgettable experience, because we said yes to everything, I mean everything--heart break, desire, challenges beyond what we thought we were capable of; and that year changed us and bonded us for life.

At twenty-six, I packed up my car and moved to Portland. I had never been before. It has been six years now and my husband and I are blissfully happy. We travel all over the world together, eat weird food, take Barre classes, plant fruit trees, and dream about the day we will get pygmy goats for our two-and-a-half-acre homestead.

My life turned out exactly the way I had always dreamed of because I said yes. I never questioned what was being thrown at me or why. I love fully, live fully, express fully, and only apologize when I really needed to. I am happy because I am fulfilled, because I didn't turn my crazy life into a negative, or blame anyone or anything for the hard parts. The hard parts were the best parts, because they taught me how to live. The hard times taught me how to fight for what was right, and what I wanted. They taught me to speak up and make my voice heard. They gave me the strength to get in a car, or a plane, and leave everything I knew. It doesn't take thirty years to grow confidence and make the life you want, it's an ever-unfolding journey, and I was happy every step of the way. Even if I didn't feel it, I found the beauty in life.

Confidence is about speaking up and saying yes to everything life puts in your way. One of my favorite quotes of all time comes from my favorite movie, *Meet Joe Black*. Cheesy as it may sound, this film continues to change my views on life, and teaches me something new every time I watch it. The quote comes at the very end, the last words of the film. The female lead asks her love: "What will we do now?" He answers her with, "It will come to us."

This is powerful on so many levels. Don't ask the questions of who, what, where, why, and how. Trust your instinct, trust your intuition, and listen to yourself. The confidence will come in the answer of giving up all responsibility. Stop over analyzing your life and just live. Give yourself permission to be confident in every decision you make. Give yourself permission to be confident. Be confident in who you are, and who you want to become. Be confident in how beautiful you truly are. If you don't want to change, don't. But if you do, don't be afraid to embrace that change. Life exists on the other side.

NOTE: If the topic of sexuality is in any way an emotional trigger, or you have been a victim of sexual assault or abuse, please proceed with caution for the remainder of this chapter.

FINDING CONFIDENCE IN OUR PRIMAL SEXUALITY

For the hundreds of female clients I have worked with in the course of my life, sex has usually been a primary motivator in their lives. Maybe they have always felt comfortable in my presence to share their most intimate selves and stories or maybe this is truly at the core of every women. As the givers of life, I feel as though women are deeply connected to their vaginal persona and root chakra whether they have explored it or not. In all of my sessions with my female clients, the want to increase libido and feel whatever their version of "sexy" is seems to always creep to the top of the list.

Even from a very young age I encouraged women and have said, "Give yourself permission to be sexual." As women, sex transcends more than we can imagine when it comes to our sense of self, our psyche, our comfort in our own bodies, and our emotional release. I know so many women that lose their libido and don't want to engage in sexual activity due to the sheer hatred they feel for their bodies. Why should we deny ourselves something that is necessary in life because of a falsely portrayed image of self? Sex and sexuality are essential to our connection to the female energy. As women, we often allow others to dictate how we feel about our bodies, but why? Why is our body another person's business? Why do they even have an opinion about our body? If we exude confidence and sexuality with our self, we can feel the immediate changes in our response to self-image. If we let insecurity rule our life we miss out, drastically.

I look at pictures of myself in my early twenties and think, "Wow I was so beautiful, why did I let other make me feel less than?" How many of you feel that way when you look back at pictures of yourself in the past? I hear it time and time again. I have even heard my mother-in-law say that when she was a teen, she thought that she was fat and ugly, and now when she looks at picture she says, "Wow I was so beautiful, I had no idea." The issue of body dysmorphia in our culture is tragic and deafening.

As I write this chapter, I have an acute awareness of my body because someone asked me this morning how much weight I think I have gained since my wedding. I said maybe ten pounds. She then asked if I owned a scale so I could keep myself on track. To keep on what track, I wondered. The only people unhappy with my body in this, or any situation, are those who are not satisfied with their own appearance. Of course, I immediately had to rewind in my head and look at this comment from an outside perspective, calm myself, and say to myself, "Hey I think you're sexy, who cares what other people think, they don't live in your body." Instead of feeling defeated and disgusted with myself, I instantly feel better. I may not physically look the way everyone thinks I should, but his or her idea of me is not what dictates my happiness or my feeling of self. Don't get me wrong, I love and adore everyone around me, but they are just as flawed as I am. Anytime someone makes me feel judged or disallowed from feeling my sexual prowess, I recalibrate and shake off their projective self-consciousness.

Once we quiet the voices and eliminate the ideas of others, we can begin to feel free. We can let the sexual tigress out.

So how do we do that? How do we recalibrate and feel sexy after being put in a box of someone else's design? It isn't easy, it takes work, but anyone can do it!

Think back to a time where you felt sexy. Don't focus too much on how you thought you looked, but rather on how you felt. What was going on? Was it an adventure of some kind? Was there a sexual experience that drove you wild? A sexy solo dance?

If we approach our sexuality from a perspective of feeling and not thought, we can understand and embrace how sexual we really are. Women live way, way, way too much inside their heads. Most women don't have sex often enough because of overthinking everything. "I'm too fat." "I have too much to do." "I don't feel sexy."

We sabotage our sexual self on the daily. Nothing gets me revved up more than sexy dancing naked in the mirror. I can feel my true, female, sexual energy in these moments. I realize how magnificent the female form is, how well we move. If we are not there yet, experiencing our body and not our idea of our body, then we can simply close our eyes and feel the movement. Feel the energy that comes from within.

I always feel sexy when I dance, because I love to dance. I have really loose hips, and I like to get down and swivel and whip them. I don't care what size they are, I'm just happy that they move! We so often take our bodies and abilities for granted. We have needs, whether or not our body looks the way we, or other people think it should. I'm talking about sexual needs!

How often do you masturbate? I try to do it as often as possible as an act of self-care. I love it! Orgasms feel amazing! I know my body so well that I can orgasm at least five times in one sitting. This is not meant to make anyone uncomfortable, these are just topics rarely discussed. We always try to hide sexuality, making it seem so perverse. Of course, you should only have sex if you want to and with someone you want to be intimate with. This isn't a way to push you beyond your limits. This is a calling to your inner sexual goddess to take charge and get exactly what you want out of life- to have it all!

Throughout most of history, men have desperately tried to silence the power of female sexuality in its natural form and fit women into their ideas of sexuality. This is the type of stuff that needs to be discussed because millions of women are walking around sexually unsatisfied, sexually shamed, and confused. Many of us are unable to explore our sexuality because we are unhappy with the way we look or have been taught that exploring our body is shameful or unnatural. We are made to believe that men will think differently of us if we express ourselves sexually. Men generate rape culture by not being aware and respectful of female sexuality.

Historically, a sexually unsatisfied woman was mistaken for and described as "hysterical" and was encouraged to go to doctors for medically induced sexual release. In an article published in *Clinical Practice and Epidemiology in Mental Health,* a few physicians describe in great medical historical detail that hysteria is one of the oldest mental disorders in women. Here is an excerpt from the article: "*Hysteria is undoubtedly the first mental disorder attributable to women, accurately described in the second millennium BC, and until Freud considered an exclusively female disease. Over 4000 years of history, this disease was considered from two perspectives: scientific and demonological. It was cured with herbs, sex or sexual abstinence, punished and purified with fire for its association with sorcery and finally, clinically studied as a disease and treated with innovative therapies. However, even at the end of the nineteenth century, scientific innovation had still not reached some places, where the only known therapies were those proposed by Galen. During the twentieth century several studies postulated the decline of hysteria amongst occidental patients (both women and men) and the escalating of this disorder in non-Western countries. The concept of hysterical neurosis is deleted with the 1980 DSM-III. The evolution of these diseases seems to be a factor linked with social "westernization", and examining under what conditions the symptoms first became common in different societies became a priority for recent studies over risk factor."*[1]

What this journal is trying to say is that the sexuality of women went undiscovered for thousands of years. Our sexual arousal and hormonal mood swings were seen as a disorder "Hysteria" and not a natural occurrence. I can't say that any of this is positive information, but it does validate the male agenda of oppression toward female sexuality. The only thanks women may have given would be to some of the physicians in the Victorian era working with female hysteria. This is how vibrators and various female oriented sex toys were born. They were "administered" during "treatments" of female hysteria. Yes, you read that correctly, doctors used to clinically masturbate women to cure them of nasty thoughts.

Some cultures today still go as far as conducting clitoridectomies, genital mutilation through the removal or circumcision of the clitoris. These are cruel and sick displays of male dominated cultures. Men did not believe women deserved the same satisfaction because until recently the female orgasm was said to not exist. Men actually said that women weren't capable of orgasms. So, if you feel as though you aren't "sexual" it may be because of millennia of bad science, dating back to the second century, oppression, brain washing, and shame.

Does that also mean our need for sexual release decreases when we are unhappy with our appearance? Absolutely not. Does that mean there is only one size a woman can be to experience her sexuality? No! Every woman is capable of sexual satisfaction and every woman, no matter her size or circumstance is deserving of sexual pleasure.

What does any of this have to do with your happy weight? If you feel comfortable in exactly who you are, including your nakedness and sexuality, you can begin to appreciate your body as a whole. You can be happy in exactly who you are. What does happiness do exactly? It disallows negative hormones from creeping in and ruining our quality of life.

Now, let's get down to the nitty gritty! I'm going to recommend a few things to activate your inner sex goddess so you can start to radiate your magnificent beauty from the inside out!

1. Write down all of the amazingly beautiful things you love about yourself. It doesn't have to be physical. Brains, wit, and positive actions of all kinds are insanely sexy.

2. Dance naked in front of a mirror. Glance at all of your glory and beauty!

3. Try something new that is sexually related, like a new form of movement or something that engages your sexual self, such as Buti Yoga or skinny-dipping!

4. Get to know your body, sexually speaking. What is it that you like? Do you know how to give yourself an orgasm? Once you are able to get outside of your head and enjoy yourself honestly, wholeheartedly, and without a negative idea of self, your vagina and inner goddess will thank you.

5. Wear something that makes you feel empowered, something that makes you feel good about yourself. It can be whatever you want, express yourself without the thoughts and opinions of others.

Now that we have all of these fun sexually invigorating tips, let's talk about how beneficial orgasms are for our overall health.

Sexual Constipation Can Be Toxic

Sexpert and world-famous vaginal weight lifter Kim Anami often speaks of the deep spiritual power the female orgasm has. She says that it is vitally necessary for women to experience a true, deep, vocal, and connected intravaginal orgasm on a regular basis.[2] If we are having unsatisfying, short, clitoral orgasms just to "get it over with," we are seriously unfulfilled in our love life, not to mention lacking access to the powerful emotion behind the full extent of the female orgasm.

Consistent sexual release has endless health benefits. Oxytocin released after the female orgasm is proven to reduce stress and create an overall feeling of wellbeing.[2] Increased endorphins can induce deeper relaxation and deeper sleep for many[3]. I myself have woken up in the middle of the night, unable to fall back asleep for various reasons, and was able to fall back to sleep after I masturbated and climaxed. It is better to use a natural approach than prescribed sleep aids, which only perpetuate health issues. Orgasms can also help to alleviate pain and strengthen neuro-positive chemicals like serotonin to enhance mood and behavior. This is all revolving around the positive chemicals released into the body and brain post orgasm.[4] I have even used orgasms to alleviate menstrual cramps!

Whether you are invoking your sexuality to build confidence or increase health benefits, it is important to engage in regular sexual activity with yourself, in a sexually driven class, or safely with a partner.

When discussing confidence, everyone will choose a different path. We all come from various backgrounds and all have different perspectives and experiences. Regardless, I encourage you to start your journey to realizing how absolutely special, unique, and powerful you are. You are capable of anything. Your body is beautiful, express it, live in it, understand it, love it.

CHAPTER 8

We Are All Melody!

by Melody Larue

This chapter will give you a peek into the struggles and success of my client, Melody LaRue, in her own words, as told to me.

U p. Down. Up. Down . . . Our circumstances and our results may differ, but I think that everyone's lives can be broken down into these simple terms. I was a relatively active child. I participated in sports and dance throughout early childhood, and as I went into my teen years, I went beyond the regular physical education classes, taking aerobics and weight training in school. I was healthy and strong, although my eating habits mirrored other teens of the 1990s: sugary cereals, fast foods, candy, Slurpees, and soda. My idea of vegetables was the french fries that came with my cheeseburger.

And then, at the age of nineteen, I had my first child. I was young and not well educated on healthy eating habits. Growing up, low-fat and no-fat foods were all the rage. We were told margarine was better than butter. Almost everything we ate was processed, fast, and convenient. After giving birth to my daughter, I moved out on my own for the first time and my three-year, emotionally abusive relationship with my child's father had ended. I had never cared for a baby before, so I changed my first diaper on the day she was born. I was learning how to care for myself and for my child at the same time. For five days I tried to nurse my daughter, but for some reason my milk never came. She would cry all day and night, so I finally caved and fed her formula. She would projectile vomit after every feeding. She screamed every time I bathed her. I cut her little finger the first time I tried to clip her nails. I became depressed. I felt like a failure of a mother and constantly wondered if I would be able to provide for her. I was overwhelmed to say the least.

This was the time my weight gain really began. Initially, my "baby weight" seemed to disappear, which tricked me into thinking that I was one of the lucky ones who could eat anything and not gain weight. I did, however, try to eat healthy. At least what I thought was healthy. I remember buying frozen vegetables with cheese sauce packets and feeling proud that I was eating healthy. I didn't have the money to buy new clothes and I couldn't quite fit into the old. I kept wearing my maternity clothes, so as I slowly started to gain weight, I didn't notice. I didn't notice until one of my roommates pointed to my stomach, and asked, "Where did that come from?" I felt defeated, so I kept eating. Around that time, my daughter's father started to come around again, and I let him. He knew how to push my buttons and he knew how insecure I was about being a mother. He used that to make me feel even worse. When my daughter was five months old, I knew something had to change.

I made the bold decision to move. I needed a clean slate, a fresh start. I left my parents and my sister, who had been my only support system, and moved to a town six hours away, a town I had never even visited, that had a college and a few acquaintances of mine. I started a new life for my daughter and for myself. I enrolled in the local community college at the age of twenty. I had an apartment and a roommate. My roommate helped with my daughter while I went to school. After a while, I started to feel better. I began to fit into my role as a mother, and although I wasn't losing the weight I had gained after my pregnancy, I wasn't gaining weight either. I wasn't eating out of sadness or loneliness anymore.

Fast forward four years, after multiple moves across the country and back, and one failed marriage, I was back on the West Coast and temporarily living with my parents. My dad got me an interview with an insurance company in his building. Soon, I was working for them, as a data entry clerk on the graveyard shift. It worked perfectly. I didn't have to hire a babysitter, since my parents were home in the evenings with my daughter. It was also the start of another few years of weight gain and unhealthy habits.

Working in a seven-story building, at night, all alone, was strange. I wasn't a great planner, and would show up for work without thinking to bring food for the night. Most nights I didn't eat at all. I'd stuff myself after work, and then sleep most of the day. Sometimes weeks would go by without me sitting down to a real meal. A few months into working for this company, I quit smoking, which led to a lot of vending machine snacking throughout my late night shifts.

I eventually started dating again, and within a year was living with my future husband. After suffering a couple of miscarriages and being told I probably wouldn't have more children, I had my second child, another girl. I didn't gain nearly as much weight as with my first, but I was a lot heavier this time around. I still hadn't tried to lose the weight I had gained with my firstborn, so I was a bit more careful with my eating habits. My food cravings were just as intense, but different.

With my first pregnancy, I craved chili cheese dogs and

Slurpees. This time around, I craved canned pineapple. What a change! I ate so much pineapple that my friends and coworkers wondered how the inside of my mouth wasn't torn apart!

Interestingly, my firstborn is a vegetarian and my second child hates anything that tastes like pineapple!

My oldest was six at this point, school age, but I decided to homeschool. My husband worked and I stayed home with our kids. My days were filled with lessons with my oldest, caring for my new baby, cleaning house, and making meals. My evenings were spent preparing lessons for the following day, and after the work was done, I watched television, and snacked. I was comfortable, happy, and felt like I was exactly where I was supposed to be in life. I was so far removed from that nineteen-year-old girl who was so frightened and unsure of herself as a mother. I had this.

As the years went by, I took care of everyone, most times forgetting to take care of myself. I remember days when I never even changed out of my pajamas. I kept myself so busy with my children that I'd forget to eat during the day. In the evenings, once the hunger hit, I'd binge until bedtime. Now, I was gaining weight, but for entirely different reasons.

For the next couple of years, I suffered several miscarriages. My husband and I wanted to have a big family, so we kept trying. The inability to carry my children to term started to weigh on me. I started to revert back to those feelings of inadequacy that I had when I was nineteen. I felt like a failure. But then, we had our miracle. When my second child was four years old, I gave birth to a boy. By this time, I was at my heaviest. I wasn't even thirty yet, and I weighed well over 200 pounds. My body was aching, I had trouble breathing, my blood pressure was high, and normal activities like playing with my children seemed daunting. This was when I had another moment of clarity, much like the feeling I had when I moved away from my family and created a new beginning.

After so many years of poor habits, I knew I needed help. I

joined a program that I thought would help motivate me and help keep me accountable. I went to the weekly meetings, I counted my points, and I kept a perfect food and exercise journal. I finally began to lose weight. I lost fifty pounds that year. I felt great and thought I had finally found something that would work for me. The following year, my husband was injured on the job. He had to have surgery and physical therapy, and wouldn't be able to work. This meant we had to give up all the extras, and we could no longer afford my weight loss program. I felt confident that I could continue to lose weight. I was tired of tracking points by this time, and thought I knew enough about food labels, healthy eating habits, and exercise to continue the journey on my own.

I was still homeschooling my children and had even started a homeschool group with other mothers. We met twice per week and did all of our own lessons and projects. When my husband was injured, I had to get a job. The only thing I really knew how to do, that would offer me flexibility, was waitressing. I thought I could work and still take care of everything else. After all, mothers are superheroes, right? We are supposed to be able to do it all without a second thought. That year I ended up with two jobs and continued to homeschool my kids. I was beyond exhausted and frustrated with the turn our lives had taken.

My weight loss halted again. I didn't gain weight, like I had before, but I was eating on the go, if at all. Most days I ate once per day. I started talking about it with some friends from work and one of them mentioned a weight loss challenge she was involved with. I wasn't sure if I could do it, because participation meant buying products and we were broke. However, there was a cash prize involved and I needed something to motivate me again. I went for it. I drank the shakes, took the vitamins, kept the food journal, and exercised every day. I won the challenge! I was inspired again.

At first, this program was perfect for me in many ways. I was always on the go and didn't have time to cook or sit down to eat. After a full day of homeschooling the kids, taking care of a baby, and then working at night, the last thing I wanted to do was prepare a meal. So, I drank shakes, sometimes up to three per day. I took a ton of supplements and when I did eat real food, it was something from the restaurant I worked at, which was loaded with vegetable oils and sodium.

I lived like this for several years and even started to find time for exercise. My oldest was a teenager and we needed to start tracking credits since she wasn't in a traditional school. She was never into dance or sports, and most beginner classes do not cater to fourteen-year-olds. I decided to enroll her in a Krav Maga class. That would give her some self-defense skills and qualified as a full PE credit. After watching her first class, I decided to join her. We had so much fun together and I started to feel healthy and strong again. At this point it wasn't about losing weight; it was about feeling good. I was so overwhelmed with working full-time, homeschooling, and having a toddler that the exercise renewed my energy. The weight loss was a bonus. Within two years, I had reached my goal and lost one hundred pounds.

Throughout all of this, I began to realize my marriage was falling apart. Before his injury, my husband worked out of town five to six days per week for several years. I had created a life that didn't really include him, not because I didn't want him involved, but because he wasn't there. I hated that most of his business was out of town. I tried to come up with ideas to make his business more local, but he wasn't receptive to them. After his injury, when he was home all day, every day, we started to realize that we had grown apart. We led separate lives for so many years that we no longer had very much in common. We tried to change that. We took swing dance lessons, went to dinner and a movie once per month, and tried to get to know each other again. It did not take long before I realized the spark was gone and it likely wasn't coming back. I still wasn't ready to give up, so I suggested marriage counseling. We tried that for a few months and then I made the most difficult decision I had ever made, and told him I wanted a divorce. Soon after, I found a house close to our neighborhood, and just as our kids and I were moving, I lost my job. It was the first time I had a place of my own, and now I was now an unemployed, single, mom.

Although the separation was difficult for us all, it made my ex-husband a better father. He was more attentive to our children, he was more involved in their lives, and he worked in town more often. After six months of living on unemployment, child support, and food stamps, I landed a job as a bartender.

Over the next two years, I worked ten-hour days, five days per week. I still tried to homeschool, but was falling behind. I couldn't keep up with it all, which led to those feelings of inadequacy that I thought had disappeared. Weren't my problems supposed to disappear once I was skinny? My ex-husband and I were fighting, and it was beginning to feel as if we'd never find a way to co-parent. I was exhausted and overwhelmed. This time, I didn't eat away my emotions. I drank them away, or tried to anyway. I knew my kids would be asleep by the time I was off work, so I'd head to my favorite bar for a drink, which most of the time, led to multiple drinks. I'd wake with hangovers and very little energy for my responsibilities. Then tragedy struck, a tragedy that blindsided us all.

My ex-husband, the father of my children, the one who raised my oldest like his own, had a heart attack at age thirty-eight. Life support kept him breathing for almost a week, but his brain never recovered from the lack of oxygen after his heart failed. We had to make the decision to take him off life support, and within ten minutes he was gone. I felt more alone than I'd ever felt. I had no idea what to do next.

My kids and I started grief counseling right away. I quit my job so that I could be with them to help them through their grief. It was the most difficult thing we could have faced. Seeing the looks of sadness every day, and hearing their cries every night was almost unbearable. I'd tell you more about those first few months if I could remember them. When I think back, it's like it was all a dream. You know those mornings when you remember everything in a dream vividly, but within a few minutes your memory becomes fuzzy and by the end of the day you can't recall any of the details? That's what it's like when you lose someone, except that when you wake, they're still gone.

The loss of my children' dad will always be a part of our everyday lives, and something none of us will ever "get over." He won't be there for high school graduations, wedding days, or to welcome grandchildren into the world. Each happy moment will always be laced with sadness. However, we needed to live again, and my therapists told me that my kids would never learn how to unless I showed them. I had to lead by example.

My oldest had graduated high school, her last two years partic-ipating in the Running Start program at our local community college, and had moved to the east coast. She had been accepted to a university there and was well on her way to living her own life. My younger two entered into public school, for the first time, as a seventh grader and a third grader. I started a new job, bartending again. Everything had changed.

I was terrified. I felt like I was going through the motions of doing everything right, but that at anytime the other shoe was going to drop. We were still in counseling, we were moving forward, we were learning how to live after this tragedy. I questioned every decision and was so scared, it was debilitating. I started having panic attacks, which I had never experienced before. I began drinking heavily again, which made the anxiety worse. I felt worse than I ever had, and not only was I suffering, but more importantly, my kids were suffering. I made excuses for myself, like "I only go out after my kids are asleep, so it's not taking time from them." Even then, I think I must've known that I was full of the proverbial "it."

We lived like this for a couple of years. I was gaining weight, slowly, but surely. I was making unhealthy choices, physically and emotionally. I began a new relationship, that was rocky at best, and when it ended, I felt like my world had fallen apart. Although there were a lot of circumstances that ended that relationship, I know I had put a lot of pressure on it. I turned it into the glue that held me together. It was easier to focus on the problems of that relationship than with my own problems stemming from my ex-husband's death. When it ended, it made me face everything all at once. I was angry, defeated, self-pitying, and I just wanted to run from it all.

I tried a couple of times to diet and exercise again, but I just wasn't inspired. I kept eating and drinking and feeling sorry for myself. I had moments of clarity that made me feel like I would motivate myself to change, like I had in the past. However, this time, I couldn't stay motivated for longer than a few days. I tried counting points again. I tried drinking shakes again. I couldn't stick to anything. The pounds started creeping up on me.

I was still angry. Angry about everything. I wallowed in it. I turned myself into a victim, who made me feel even more pathetic, which led to more unhealthy behaviors. I had dug myself into a hole. A hole that was full of desperation and fear. A hole I felt stuck in, with no way out.

I tried to hide my drinking from my kids. I know I did a poor job of it; they are smart children who know when their mother isn't quite right. One night, of which the details are too humiliating to admit, my kids were trying to get a hold of me. I wasn't answering my phone. They became frightened and called work. I had left work hours before, so now my co-workers were worried. They began calling the friends they knew I went out with on a regular basis. By the time I finally stumbled home, almost everyone I knew had been trying to locate me. I was devastated and so angry with myself. My children only had one parent left. And that parent had completely fallen apart before their eyes.

This was my wake-up call. My kids deserved better. They were struggling and watching me struggle was not something they needed. I had to figure this out, if not for me, for them. I was living in a place called rock bottom. I had been close to this place before, but managed to drive by and never stop. This time was different. I knew I had to ignore my negative self-talk, I had to quit feeling sorry for myself, and I had to quit sabotaging myself.

It was around this time that a good friend of mine decided to move to Los Angeles. She wasn't quite sure how she was going to do it, but she was determined. I thought this would be the perfect opportunity for me to get away, to clear my head. I offered to drive her, so we loaded up my car and headed south. We spent two days driving and then I spent another two with her in her new home. It was hard to part ways, but I knew I needed to be alone to gather my thoughts and take a long, hard look at my life. I drove up the coast of California, with my windows down, and my music loud. I stopped in beautiful towns, walking barefoot on their beaches, and dining in their restaurants. I quite literally wandered their streets aimlessly, with no one destination in mind. It was exactly what I needed. I returned home with a new energy, motivated to get everything on track.

I began to create my own happiness. I started leaving the bar after work, and I stopped going out on my days off. I reconnected with an old friend who moved a little over an hour away. Her and I have dinner every month or so, dinner that doesn't include cocktails. I started getting massages every six weeks to help with my aching muscles. I began cooking, a lot. I'd gather recipes for the week one evening and the next morning would buy the groceries needed. I'd cook the entire day and eat the food all week. I started cooking for friends too. I prepared meals two weeks in a row for my friend who had a baby. I started reading again, an old passion from my childhood. I hadn't read a book from cover to cover in a long time. I even co-created a book club with a couple of friends. I put on dresses and red lipstick and even when I didn't believe it, I told myself I was beautiful. It took about six months after that dreaded night when my kids couldn't find me, but I was feeling like myself again. I wasn't truly there yet, but I was moving forward. I was a better mother, a better friend, and a better me.

This is when life tested me, again. I reconnected with the

man from my last relationship, at first, just in friendship. He was sick; the kind of sick where one might not recover. He spent nearly a month in the hospital. During that time, I had trouble leaving his side, terrified that each visit would be our last. For one fleeting moment, old thoughts started to creep back. My inner monologue was what you might imagine: negative and self-pitying. I knew the drill. But then, unlike before, I stopped myself.

During his hospital stay we had hours-long conversations about everything under the sun. We laughed a lot, even when the timing seemed inappropriate. We watched horrible reality television shows. We dined on takeout because hospital food is worse than a middle school cafeteria. We spent more time together in thirty days of visiting hours than we did the entire span of our nine-month relationship. He swears to this day that my visits are what kept him going, and that our laughter helped to heal him. That may be somewhat true, but he has strength like I've never seen. He did all the heavy lifting; I was just there to hold his hand.

After he was healthy enough, he was finally able to leave the hospital. However, my health had started to deteriorate. I had gained the hundred pounds back that I lost years prior, but this time I was forty. My hands and feet were in so much pain on a daily basis, that I could barely walk after work, or make my hands into fists. It was getting worse by the day. So much worse that I thought I'd have to find another line of work. Ten-hour shifts on my feet were almost impossible now. My weight felt different too. I felt puffy and swollen, almost like when I was pregnant, but worse.

That is when I went to see Daniele. I didn't know much about nutrition therapy, but at that point, I was willing to try anything. After what my family and I had just been through with my boyfriend's hospital stay, I knew I needed to make health my number one priority.

I learned a lot during my initial meeting with Daniele. I was overwhelmed with all of the new information, but it made so much sense that I knew it was something I needed to do. Daniele was able to address some of the causes of my joint pain and my weight gain almost immediately. I had just assumed my problems were all related to being overweight. It turned out, my weight gain was caused by some of the dysfunction in my body, which was related to foods I was consuming that did not agree with my body.

When Daniele told me that I had nightshade intolerance, my first question was, "What the hell is a nightshade?"

She replied, "Tomatoes, all peppers, white, red, and purple potatoes, and eggplant."

I had no idea that any of these foods had anything in common. I also had no idea that it was going to be so difficult to eliminate these foods. My favorite foods are Mediterranean, Thai, and Mexican, all of which contain some sort of tomato and/or pepper.

Gluten was another factor, but I wasn't too worried because I've never been a huge bread eater. I wasn't worried until I began to learn how many things contain gluten. It's not just about the bread!

I was focused and I was determined that first month. I had a huge support system, which included my kids, my boyfriend, Daniele (who I met with every week those first few months), and my chefs at work. I began experimenting with different foods I hadn't really tried before. I found a lot of things I loved, and others not so much. I was eating breakfast, lunch, dinner, and snacks in between. I was never hungry. My body was full of healthy fats, protein, vegetables, and fruits. I researched the things that Daniele taught me about in our weekly meetings. I learned about gut health and its link to our brain (a subject dear to me as I had a great-grandmother with Alzheimer's disease and I have a grandmother living with dementia). I added pickled vegetables into my routine. I took my supplements, including magnesium, multivitamins, amino acids, and eliminated alcohol.

By the end of that first month, I felt incredible. My joint pain had improved significantly, and that puffy, swollen feeling had all but gone away. It was working. I wasn't counting points, I wasn't drinking shakes, I wasn't on a diet. I was living. And as a bonus I lost some weight.

How much? I have no idea. I don't weigh myself. That number doesn't matter and it doesn't deserve my attention. I don't need a scale to tell me when I'm losing weight or when I'm feeling good. I know because my clothes fit different and I have more energy. What I can tell you is that one year later, I am three sizes smaller, I hiked almost eleven miles in Glacier National Park this summer, and each week I go on five- to seven-mile walks with a friend. After a ten-hour shift on my feet, I don't go straight to bed. And I continue to tell myself that skinny does not equal happy, but strong and healthy does.

There are several reasons I decided to tell my story, the most important being that everyone has stress, everyone has hardships, everyone fails, and everyone succeeds. We are each on a different path. They lead us in different directions, but we must always remember that the journey is the most important part. An old friend of mine once said, "It's not about the big ending, it's about all the smalls along the way." I had to teach myself that no matter what is happening in my life, my health is important. Without it, there isn't anything else.

If I eat something that isn't in my plan, I don't call it a cheat; I call it an indulgence and move on with my day. Here's an example. My son is learning to cook. He wanted to make a recipe that came in a monthly subscription, called "Hellboy Hotwings and Anti-Potato Salad." It was gluten free, but definitely NOT nightshade free. You know what I did? I ate the dinner he wanted to prepare for us, and I enjoyed every bite, guilt-free. I was able to do that because I know that tomorrow I won't have night-shades. I know what I'm doing now. I plan and I prepare, but I also indulge when it feels right to do so. I learned to stop beating myself up.

I have created a life that makes me happy. I surround myself with supportive, positive people. I stop and smell every rose. Last year, my boyfriend and I were driving through western Colorado and southern Utah. We stopped at almost every viewpoint and some spots in between. We wanted each one to last forever because we didn't think it could get any better than it already had. But each corner we turned was more beautiful than the last. This is my life now. Sometimes I am up, and sometimes I am down. Regardless, it's all beautiful.

CHAPTER 9
Selfishness: The Art Of Setting Boundaries

The need to please everyone pleases no one, if you are not pleased with yourself, you will never find true happiness.

B oundaries are extremely important for everything: stress management, toxic relationships, personal growth, energy conservation, and our overall health and wellbeing. Some people see boundaries as selfish. Selfishness is such a dirty word. People use it all of the time to describe situations they don't completely understand. It is a judgment word used by those who don't have the capacity to see a person through that person's eyes. People have so many expectations about how a person is "supposed" to be. I am over people thinking that others are supposed to be a certain way. Leave people alone, and let them live their lives. Are we so bored that we need to be concerned with everyone else's lives?

This is what I think every time a person has an expectation

for me or someone tries to micromanage my life. Since becoming an adult I have had this amazing ability to cut people out if I ever felt them trying to control me with their own selfish agenda. In this chapter, I am going to help you understand how that works.

I have met so many women over the years that don't make changes in their health because of the influence of others: others' needs, wants, impressions, and ideas. It is all the garbage that doesn't matter when it comes to you taking care of yourself. So many times I have heard, "I can't say no, it's rude." Rude to whom? And why is that your responsibility?

I have heard, "But that's just the way they are." No! Any time a family member or significant other has tried to say anything about my body or food choices that is negative, I throw it straight back in their face. It is not love or care if someone is judging you. It is not compassion or understanding if someone is forcing something on you or trying to tell you how to be. It is not friendship or companionship if someone is micromanaging everything you do. You are who you are and should be loved for exactly that. Your food choices or appearance should never be a part of the equation. If you are hurting yourself or others in a direct way, that's a different story. But if your mother is telling you that you are fat and you shouldn't be eating something, tell her to mind her own damned business.

When someone is judging you it always comes back to his or her personal issues. They are projecting their own insecurities by trying to cut you down and bring you to whatever miserable level they are living on at that time in their life.

But being honest with people is hard! Telling them exactly how we feel can be paralyzing. I have so many friends that don't tell their families anything about themselves because of that fear. This type of honesty can often leave us with a huge "vulnerability hangover." This term is something Bréne Brown defines as the feeling that we get after revealing our truth.[1] We become hyper aware of ourselves, fear not being liked, or fear judgment itself.

But how can we break free of the imprisonment people put

on us if we don't set boundaries? How can we see controlling people for who they are? How can we stand comfortably in our truth?

What I am trying to encourage here is: Don't waste time worrying if people don't like you, and don't engage in negative conversation unless your morals are challenged. And if your morals are challenged, stand up for yourself, and for what you believe in!

Stop Being Polite And Awaken Your Voice

As women, we are seen as cute and tiny in a proverbial sense. If we act weak, we will be seen as weak and the idea of who we are will be silenced or put into a cute, tiny box. I grew up receiving no respect from others because they thought that *innocent* was tattooed on my forehead. I am by no means innocent, weak, or incapable. Some people instantly think that because we have a vagina that we are completely useless or helpless. But we, as women, are the complete opposite. Not only are we capable, strong, creative, and resourceful, if we stand strong, together we can rule the world.

A vulnerability hangover should never be a part of the equation because as women we should be steadfast in who we are, who we see ourselves as, and what we believe in. We should always be made to feel as though our thoughts, feelings, and self is worthy. If we feel a vulnerability hangover, we are feeling guilt and shame, we are invalidating whom we are, we are saying to ourselves, "hey, everything you did today is wrong, and others are judging you."

Is this what you want other women to feel after having a conversation with you? No? So let's look at that from a personal perspective and believe that we are worthy of the conversation.

Finding your happy weight is not about religion, it is not about God, it is not about man vs. woman, or about societal roles. Finding your happy weight is not meant to challenge your moral compass or belief system; it is about you being heard. It is about eliminating walls built around social constructs, eliminating judgment, eliminating the idea that there is one way to be, or one way to exist.

If we truly understand what it is to be heard, loved, understood, validated, and respected, we will feel that sense of wholeness and completeness. Happy weight is about disregarding another person's opinion about what we put in our mouth, how we decided to look, or how we choose to walk our personal path to wellness. There is no THEM in YOU. That is not how life works. No matter what we believe, people forcing their ideas on us is destructive.

Boundaries are the key to freedom and if people don't respect your boundaries, you should remove them from your life.

I do it, and it feels great every time! Not a single person on this planet is allowed to make us a slave to them in any way, shape, or form. Not mentally, emotionally, or physically. When someone has an expectation of us, his or her disappointment can be defining. Having a constant need to please another person is excruciating. It is not worth our time.

In my life I am a prisoner to no one. I say yes a lot, only because I am given so many beautiful opportunities to experience people and life. I say no to the people that serve no purpose or the situations I have no desire to partake in.

If peer pressure still exists in your life and you are over the age of sixteen, it's time to own your worth. It's time to realize that you are capable of so much more.

Right now, some of you may be thinking, what do boundaries have to do with weight? I personally think they have everything to do with it. For example, some of you don't know how to say no to going out to happy hour, dinner, or drinks with a friend regardless of your triggers with food or alcohol that will inevitably derail your path to reaching health and wellness goals.

A good boundary would be meeting for a hike, walk, or yoga class instead of always meeting for "food centered" activities.

Learning to say no to people and establishing boundaries can save us from the habits that are keeping us in an unhealthy state.

Another example of setting boundaries is when a friend invites you over for dinner without discussing the contents of the meal, bring your own food, it's not rude if it saves you from being sick for several days because you are more concerned with the hosts opinion of you than maintaining your health.

Like I said earlier, as women we have the power of voice, we have the power to control how we see ourselves, how we live our lives, what we choose to make of our choices.

Ownership is at the root of boundaries. If we take ownership over our decisions regarding our body and our health we can make unbelievable strides toward our happy weight. Say yes to the things we want and no to the things we don't. Don't be bullied or reduced into making choices that are not ultimately our own.

All of my life people have said before I even order my food, "Oh that sounds like a Daniele meal." I'm not sure what that means, but so many times I have been subconsciously programmed to order whatever that meal was despite my intentions or personal choice, because a single comment made me identify with that. We are so easily seduced into an idea by another person. We fall victim to it. But we are conscious and have thought, and can decide the type of food we want to eat. We should do it and not be controlled by others.

Don't be controlled by your past. Don't be controlled by an idea you may have of your past self, if you choose to not see yourself as the old you. Be the person you want to be and demand respect with boundary language that makes statements about what you really want!

Saying you "can't" have something, gives a third party the control over your choices. Saying you chose not to, gives you ownership and solidifies the boundary.

The next time a person tries to impose their idea of what you should eat on you, you can respond with statements such as these:

- "I am going to eat that because I want to, because it brings my body nourishment, because I don't want to put harmful foods into my body."

- "I am **not** going to eat that, because it doesn't bring my body nourishment, because I don't want to put harmful foods into my body."

- "No thank you, I am choosing not to eat _____. I am focusing on my personal health."

- "I have chosen to no longer eat that/those type(s) of food(s) for the betterment of my health."

- "I would appreciate it if you would be so kind as to no to impose your choices on me, I am choosing to be more mindful with my own personal health and body, so my food choices may change, please respect that."

- "That sounds great, but I am trying out some new choices with my health, would you mind doing a non-food centered activity?"

These of course are just examples of using boundary language. In this way, you are asking others to respect your choices and taking ownership with pride. Making these statements disallows the person from imposing their idea, because you have ultimately made the best choice for you!

CHAPTER 10
Find Your Tribe, Find Yourself

Knowing yourself is the beginning of all wisdom.

Aristotle

Body image is the outer layer of seeking acceptance. There is also this element of acceptance from within: your personality and who you perceive yourself to be. Everyone on this planet, male, female, black, white, short, tall, gay, trans, we all at some point or another seek connection. We want to be like those around us, that's why we take on the traits of our parents, our friends, our lovers. We are constantly seeking acceptance. We feel that if we are accepted then we will finally "fit in." Fitting in, is the innate need to belong to a tribe. We are community driven beings; it is engrained in what we are. For the sake of getting scientific, this instinct is survival based, primal. We join a tribe for protection, safety, shelter, family, survival, and so on. We have a biological imperative to continue our existence, and an inner drive to ensure the survival of our species[1]. Today we are so populated that the number of tribes to subscribe to are endless. What does this have to do with finding yourself and being happy?

If we don't first seek our true tribe, we may never find ourselves. For example, I thought that my family was my tribe, but I am very different from them. I got a great education of how people could be different when I moved to Norway, but it wasn't until I moved to China and found my tribe that I discovered who I really was and what I was truly capable of. It was my dear friend, Rich, who told me years ago that he couldn't wait to meet the future me because I would become one of the coolest people he would ever meet. I thought at the time, "What an odd thing to say." It wasn't meant to be negative, it simply was that I hadn't met myself yet. I had just met my tribe and through my experience with them I was going to eventually meet the true me.

How could I know that these people were my tribe? For starters, they never judged me, not once. It was the most bizarre and beautiful experience of my life. These people had opinions, we all do, but they let me be myself. They let me figure out who I even was. They pushed my limits, said insanely inappropriate things, and got drunk all without making me feel like I always had to keep it together. They let me experience life. I wasn't constantly afraid of losing the approval of everyone around me because they were always going to be my friends. They never hid anything from me, never lied to me, and never made me feel as though I was not worthy enough to hold their secrets. They were also unapologetically themselves. As I write this, ten years later, we are all still as close as we were. We talk weekly, even though none of us live in the same city. We even all have matching tattoos that we got on my wedding night. That was a conscious decision that all of us made in our thirties. We are branded for life. From an anthropological standpoint, this is something many tribes did to represent themselves. Since China, I have found myself, along with many other amazing tribe members along the way, who have become my extended family.

What does finding our tribe have to do with finding our

happy weight? A lot! It's a huge part of accepting who we are, who we are becoming, or who we want to be. We don't choose where we are born, what kind of life we are raised into, or what our parents have decided for us.

Don't stress about where you are now or how you have been living, that is only a blip, only a millisecond in your life. Like I said once before, every second in your life is a chance to choose something different. Finding your tribe helps you find your happy weight because your tribe is comprised of people that push you to be you, to be the best version of you. They don't judge, they encourage. They don't tear you down, they only give you constructive criticism to steer you in the right direction. What is the right direction? It is what you want it to be!

I always wanted to live in a world where everyone was loved and allowed to be exactly who they wanted to be. I love everyone! That is no joke. Every person I meet I love, especially when they are completely open! If you're gay, bisexual, or transgender, I love you. If you're Muslim, Christian, or Hindu, I love you. If you're disfigured or disabled, I love you. If you're HIV positive, suffering from Lyme disease or multiple sclerosis, I love you. If you have piercings, body modifications, and tattoos all over your body, I love you! No matter what you weigh or what you look like, I love you! Be you and I will love you!

FIND TEAM YOU!

These are the qualifications for finding your tribe: find a group of people that are on your team, your own personal group of cheerleaders. Find people that love you, NO MATTER WHAT.

Once the pressure of feeling like you have to be a certain way is gone, the real you will magically appear, and start to develop, relax, and form into who you always knew you wanted to be.

If you live in a city, work a job in an office, have a network of people that you don't really click with, and you are always called to the outdoors, find a tribe that lives for the outdoors! I understand that there is fear surrounding meeting new people and trying new situations, but what will happen if you never try? You will continue to feel unfulfilled and continue to live a life that isn't really you. Remember the chapter about vulnerability? If you don't put yourself out there, you will never know what life can be like.

What Is A Tribe, Really?

Do we now know what a tribe is? Maybe? Maybe not? Let's clarify a little. A tribe is a group of people that have similar interests, however big or small. My tribe is a group of people that subscribe to the term *wanderlust*. Merriam-Webster defines *wanderlust* as: a strong desire to travel[2]. As individuals, my tribe has lived and traveled all over the world, or has the desire to. Our cross-cultural needs began early in our lives and some of us experienced travel at a very young age. We lust for change, experience, culture, and education in an anthropological sense. Are we all the same? Absolutely not! If you lined us all up in terms of education, profession, and background, we could not be more different. But that's not what a tribe is about. It's about accepting each other's differences, encouraging them, and a common love and lust for life.

There Is No One Right Answer

For you, the answer could be scrapbooking, cycling, card games, volunteering, language, politics, science, innovation, hiking, or sports. There is no right or wrong tribe; there is only what fits you! This isn't about outdoing, or being better, worse, or more valuable. This is about finding a group of people that you can't live without; people you admire and grow with. It is about finding a group where you always feel safe, and can be whomever you want to be.

Finding your tribe does require one specific thing: the willingness to change. You can't set out to find your tribe, finding yourself in the process, if you are not willing to let go of the idea of the way everything is supposed to be. If you approach this with a closed mind and with no comfort in the process of change, it might backfire.

This isn't meant to scare you. I'm simply trying to prepare you for the reality. If you are not vulnerable and open, it will be hard for your tribe to connect with you. They won't understand why you are there. Just put yourself out there and see what happens, you might surprise yourself!

Examining The Process Of Change

For some, change is too hard. It is a very vulnerable process. When we find it hard to change, it is usually due to lack of confidence in the idea of the change itself, however that manifests. If we lack the confidence in a decision and become overly aware of our insecurities, we will never be able to embrace the experience unfolding around us. Failure to make changes sets us on a path of thinking we can never accomplish anything. We enter this continuous cycle of thinking it will be different every time, yet we sabotage ourselves. One definition of insanity is doing the same thing twice and expecting a different result. How do we think we will go further than before if we are approaching the problem in exactly the same way? Discovering one's self and being dedicated to the ongoing process of growth and progress is characteristic of a woman that is capable of change. We have this ability inside ourselves; we just haven't exercised this muscle yet.

Exercising Intuition

Women have this incredible gift called intuition. We are born with an outstanding ability to feel things in our "gut." These gut feelings are a form of innate intelligence that some of us may have lost. In conversation I have heard over and over, "I knew it was a bad idea" or "I had a bad feeling about that." We have these very real, definitive radars, which we have lost the ability to use. So many times in my own life I have known the answer to something but lacked the confidence to stay steadfast in my beliefs. I have been wrong in relationships, friendships, actions, and decisions. So often we deny ourselves the satisfaction of what we feel to be true because we aren't confident in who we are. It is imperative to establish some sort of confidence in our self and in the idea of change before we seek out our tribe. If we are insecure about any ideas we have, we may end up following what everyone else wants to do and never develop into who we are meant to be. No one likes a people pleaser. Living a life of pleasing others pleases no one. People pleasers are the doormats of life. Stronger, more confident people steamroll people pleasers. It's so painful to watch. If we are able to say, "Yes, I like to do this," and, "No, I don't like to do that," with complete honesty, that is confidence. When we have ownership over an answer we become more and more confident with every statement.

It's okay if you don't know what you like or dislike. You may not be aware of the real you yet. There is an equal amount of confidence in not knowing the answer. You just have to express your not knowing and feel good about it. You are not weak or stupid if you don't know the answer to something. Not everyone knows the answer to everything, and no one likes a know-it-all. Don't mistake that attitude for confidence. Being a know-it-all reeks of insecurity. Why would someone need to prove something to you if they were confident in who they are? Exactly. They aren't.

Think about it honestly. How many times have you been swayed by someone else's opinion? When was the last time you made a choice based on what you really wanted because you knew what you wanted?

I find that one of the biggest issues with women in relationships is that they lack the understanding of themselves and what they want out of life. They end up getting divorced and burning bridges. My marriage is 100 percent egalitarian because no one tells me what to do. I do whatever I want and have no regrets, because I know who I am, and I know I'm a good person. I am always concerned for the feelings of others and make decisions based on what works for me. This makes me sound high maintenance, but it is actually the opposite. I'm easier to deal with, because I know what I want.

Getting to know yourself takes risk and dedication, but I promise you it is worth every bit. Some people call it soul searching. I think this is very accurate because you are certainly searching for something. This something already exists inside of you, and the journey brings this part out of you. It's like this version of you has always existed, you just need to peel back some layers to uncover the beauty of your deepest self.

Personally, I have always been outwardly gentle and calm. People typically categorize me as a kind and giving person. However sweet that may seem, I'm so much more than that. I feel very differently about the person I know to be my true self. I'm stubborn, opinionated, loyal, loving, and have a very sharp tongue. I'm complicated. I solve my own problems. I make my own way. Kind and giving makes me sound like Mother Teresa. She was an incredible human that did amazing things. I am just not that. I don't pretend I am something I will never be. This might also make me sound as though I am not trying to live my life as a good person, but that isn't the case either. I am constantly trying to do better, to be better. But I don't lie about who I am and I don't make excuses. So often women falsify their portrait to save face or keep up with the Joneses. I refuse to care what people think of me.

At the end of this life, we become worm food. We are organic matter that has a shelf life, an expiration date. Some may live once, some again, some go to heaven, and whatever we believe is our choice. The truth is, no matter how much conviction we have, we have no idea what is going to happen. So why are we wasting our time being something we're not?

I love what I look like because I know who I truly am. I know my true self and am acutely aware of what I am capable of. I don't apologize for who I am or for what I need to do to be fulfilled. Don't you want to feel the same way about yourself?

The Reality Check

If we are realizing now that we are not who we truly are or who we want to be, then we need help to get there. Being severed from who we really are is an uncomfortable place to be. To not be our true self is to deny all of those in our life any form of transparency.

I have friends that won't tell their parents and friends their deepest secrets because they are afraid what people will think of them. They fear that their life will be forever changed, and that they will never have a glimmer of the normalcy they think they have now. How uncomfortable it must be for them to hide who they are. At one point in my life I allowed others to make decisions for me because of fear. I didn't want to hurt anyone else's feelings and wanted everyone to be happy. This developed a very unhealthy side of me that my husband and Reiki master now refer to as my dynamite. I would push my feelings down until I couldn't any longer, at which point I would destroy everything related to that issue and then make it all disappear, never to be seen again. That is not a good way to live life.

Communication, clarity, stance, and boundaries are the best way to conduct issues and relationships. Without those four important factors, we have nothing. The fear sets in and we do not make our needs known. In the end, we never truly understand who we are or what we are capable of.

The Four Acts Of Understanding

With communication, we find our voice for the first time. We realize that once our truth is said, it's really not that scary. Eventually this grows clarity. Clarity is the moment where everything our instincts have been telling us becomes reality. It is clear and true. When we find clarity, we grow our stance. Stance is our root. It is our ground and our foundation. Without this we don't have a platform to understand ourselves, we don't have a home base in our minds that helps us to stay the course. If we don't have stance we will revert back into who we once were. When we have established our stance, we can start to make boundaries.

Setting boundaries is a topic that appears over and over in this book, because they are very significant when it comes to change and standing your ground in your new choices. Boundaries are insanely important in this life. Boundaries are also something people will struggle with until the end of time.

Boundaries are not difficult to set if you have accomplished the first three acts, which will be described below. They are simply difficult to keep presenting to people over and over again.

Most people don't understand boundaries because they don't understand why you won't do everything they want you to do. People are needy and they don't like rules, and when you set a rule for them they get uncomfortable. Their feelings are hurt. This is because most people don't exercise the four acts. They instead become children that need to be coddled. They won't respect your boundaries until they are emotionally intelligent enough to understand them. When you are not offered the respect you deserve you can offer compassion with an altruistic intention, but at the end of the day, you need to do what is best for you.

Rest assured, in time you will make friends that have heathy boundaries too, and one day life will seem very easy.

The following Acts of Understanding yourself are to be taken in stride. Listen to them, understand them, digest them. They are quick to read, but take time to fully comprehend.

Act I: Establishing Communication

Communication is the first act of understanding our self. Through communication we find our voice, we solidify and validate how we truly feel on the inside, and we find conviction.

The word 'conviction' has so many meanings, but is always so finite, so definitive. To have conviction over something makes that one thing tangible, almost like it's alive. An idea that is alive can almost be touched, and can absolutely be felt deep within us.

The best example of finding our voice and establishing conviction through communication would be making a statement. It could be as simple as, "I am a wanderluster, who doesn't want children." This is a true statement for me that can be hard for people to digest that don't know me. It suggests to them that I am selfish and inconsistent, a real "fly by the seat of my pants" kind of gal. Is this true? No, but this is what judgmental people who aren't comfortable in their own lives think. This is how we become fearful to speak our truth, we are welcomed with judgement that is fueled by ignorance. What happens to a person that experiences this? They begin to retreat and regret making themselves heard. There is no foul in someone not having children and deciding to travel instead. There is no harm in living the life you ultimately want to live. If you want to live in the same town you grew up in and have 100 children, it shouldn't matter to anyone. The decisions you make in this life, are yours and yours alone. No one person has the right to tell you how to live your life. Speaking your truth will set you free.

"I crave adventure," "I am happy being single", "I want to go back to school." These are true statements that may be hard for some to voice for fear of judgment. So often do we as women, silence ourselves, in fear that we are not worthy of who we are, or what we want out of life.

These are simple examples. Some examples of exercising your voice may be much more complicated or even simpler. Some are as simple as wanting a tattoo, or dying your hair purple. Others are as complicated as quitting a job you don't like, or coming out of the closet.

What does your voice sound like? What statements are you ready to make? What are you so afraid of? What is holding you back?

Establish communication no matter where you are in your journey and make your needs known!

ACT II: FINDING CLARITY

Clarity hits us like a bus. It comes to us like a swift kick to the brain. Some refer to it as an "aha" moment or an epiphany. It's when we have finally made statements that ring true to our inner voice and we see ourselves for the first time.

I specifically remember what it was like to see myself for the first time. I was living in Beijing, twenty-two years old, and full of life. It may have been the fact that I was in a foreign country or that my parents were 6,000 miles away. Whatever the reason, it was liberating. My tribe surrounded me, people that loved me for who I was, respected my beliefs, didn't judge me, and didn't hide things from me. We were fearless, loyal, and a chosen family.

I think the fact that my tribe challenged me, on a daily basis, to voice my opinions and grow my sense of self, made it impossible not to be free and clear. They didn't make my mind up for me. I owe particular thanks to my dormmates at the time, Jeanne and Blair, for helping me to understand what personal space was and define my first real set of boundaries.

Clarity comes to us after a perfect set of circumstances arise. It is a feeling of inhibition and complete freedom. We don't necessarily need people to get us there, they are just a support system.

If you don't currently have a support system, find one. They are everywhere. If you don't know where to start, MeetUp.com is an amazing platform for every type of hobby. If you don't see a group on there that interests you, you can create your own. And if you want to go it alone, by all means, do! Denying the basic human right to BE YOURSELF is the punishment of not following through on gaining clarity. Life will always be complicated, but when we find clarity, there is so much beauty in that complication, it leads us to where we a meant to be. Go find it, it's waiting for you!

Act Iii: Taking A Stance

You have arrived at the third act of finding yourself. You have established a clear line of communication, used your voice, and have spoken your peace. You have found clarity, and have realized that your changes are making life clearer and you're feeling freer with each passing day. Now it is time to take a stance and solidify your foundation. Find conviction in your beliefs in life. You have decided to follow your heart, now you must stand up for what you believe to be true in order to bring ultimate happiness into your life.

Taking a stance and finding conviction can be hard, especially when others heavily influence us. Sometimes opinionated people are annoying, so we think, "I don't want to be perceived like that." We don't have to be. We don't need to shout at everyone we meet. That's not what this is about. We are not trying to find our self so we can convert others. This is about us, not them.

Don't try to drag someone else on the journey with you. The friends I made were a support system, not my teammates or partners. You can only truly find yourself if you do all of this for you and only you. Don't ever take a stance for something because you think you are supposed to, or that you should, or that it will make so-and-so happy. Live your own life.

On the other hand, there is nothing wrong with being flexible and understanding. We are not talking about compromise here. I love compromise. The art of two different opinions coming together and making a sweet baby of equality is amazing. It teaches us how resilient and capable humans are. We're not talking about that. We are talking about formulating our own idea of what we know to be true for ourselves.

Taking a stance can be physical, by joining a volunteer group that makes your heart sing, or it can be metaphysical, setting on a spiritual journey to reach your nirvana. Whatever and however your stance manifests itself into is in your hands. I take a stance every day by waking up knowing that I am exactly where I have always wanted to be and I do whatever it takes to stay in that space. I live in the place I love, I am married to my best friend, I talk about nutrition and wellness with every new person I meet, I make my friends and family a priority, and I work my ever-loving heart out. I work hard and have a ton of fun doing it. I am fulfilled. Are you fulfilled? Are you lying to yourself or do you stand in your truth? Take a stance, stand tall, be YOU!

Act Iv: Setting Boundaries

I highlight boundaries mainly because they are one of the hardest things to keep in perpetual motion and can often cause conflict. Boundaries are classified as clear lines we make to separate ourselves from others and to define our comfort levels. We obviously won't be comfortable enough to make these happen until we have fully exercised the first three acts.

Boundaries make us uncomfortable if we don't fully understand them. A perfect example is when one person may use physical touch to interact and communicate, while another person may find touch incredibly uncomfortable. We are all connected energetically, but that doesn't mean we are all the same.

For me, boundaries are incredibly important and something I still struggle with. I have a hard time finding energetic balance. I make myself too available. I allow anyone and everyone to probe me for questions whenever they choose. I do this to make sure I am being of service to clients, friends, and family. I love helping people; it's my ultimate gift and my likely downfall.

Is it appropriate to provide this kind of availability or transparency? No. It's completely inappropriate, but I feel obligated. I say nothing. Like most hardworking people pleasers, I feel obligated to my responsibilities.

What's my take away from this? Maybe I need to have an email-only communication stream. No texting. But is it that easy? Where do I draw the line, and will it cause everything I have built to fall apart? Of course not. Everything will work out so much better, and I won't be drained all the time. Clearly I have at least one boundary left on my to-do list.

Ten years ago I had over fifty boundaries that needed to be set for different reasons and different people. I have come a long way. This process is never going to be perfect and I will always be presented with new scenarios or new personalities to deal with.

The idea here is not to say that I will streamline all of this and come out perfect. I may, however, become the perfect version of myself. I can honestly say that the world I live in now is the polar opposite to the world I lived in a decade ago. Baby steps, my friend, baby steps.

Are you now clear on what boundaries are? If not, think of it this way: If something makes you uncomfortable, you have boundaries. Sometimes you want to be a little uncomfortable in life, to not shut everything out and close off doors to experience. But boundaries can also be life changing. For instance, if you are in a committed relationship and your significant other has insecurities about you spending time with someone that could potentially derail your relationship, you set boundaries that work for you both. Or you have a family member that likes to feed you every time you come to visit despite your new style of eating; you then tell them no. That is another example of setting boundaries. Boundaries are invisible support systems we put in place to help us understand ourselves better, and to make people aware of what is okay and what isn't. Don't be afraid to tell another person what makes you happy, don't live in a prison of discomfort.

At the end of the day, there are boatloads of possibilities. It is up to you to decide what you face in your life and what boundaries you need to set.

FINDING CONNECTION TO OTHERS

Hopefully after some time using these exercises, you are able to start to develop You 2.0. Some of you may have found your tribe along the way, and some may still feel a little in the dark.

Loneliness is a horrible feeling when you are trying to make changes in your life. You may begin to regret your decision if you don't find some form of community. I mentioned before that you can join Meet Ups or find local chapters, groups, or clubs. If you are too nervous to meet people in person for the first time, join an online group. I do it all the time. I probably belong to more groups than I need to, ha! In this day and age, it can seem easier for people to connect online, and if you are one of those people, use it to your advantage.

Once you have connected with a few people and have shared personal stories, those people become a part of your story. I have one person in particular that found me on my Facebook page a while back and started asking me questions about her health. After months of exchanging messages, she found that the life she was living was not one she wanted. She eventually went through all of the acts I talk about here and found herself moving to another state just to gain perspective. She now has greater clarity, a louder voice, firmer boundaries, and is happier in her skin. We even spent a day together, having never met before, and it was lovely. She had, for the first time in a long time, found a member of her tribe. She made the leap and didn't look back. Was it uncomfortable at times? Yes. Does she regret it? Not for a second.

FINDING CONNECTION TO NATURE

We can go on walks every day and never be connected to the landscape we are in. As organic beings, we have an innate need to get back to basics. We are a combination of all four elements. Knowing this to be true, it makes me sad to think that people spend all of their time indoors. How do we know if our soul is connected to the world, if fake light, concrete, and plastic floors, surround us all day? We are like caged animals that have been domesticated so that we have forgotten who we really are. We are primal. We need to be connected to the earth in order to thrive. Every single centenarian culture (people who live to be one hundred and older) around the world spends a majority of their life outdoors.[3]

In Norway, recess is not cancelled if there is heavy rain or snow. Instead, they let their children play in the wide range of Mother Nature. They understand their primal obligation. We are only connected if we are a part of the natural world and our community.

I have never found more happiness or been healthier than when I have been in nature. It is borderline erotic. The grass between my toes, the water in my hands, the wind in my hair, the sun on my face, or the sound of rain falling in my ear. It is so melodic that I become hypnotized by its beauty and grandeur. That is why we call her Mother: She gives us life.

Americans have surrendered not to Mother Nature, but to her nasty uncle "the Machine." This machine is instant gratification, more of everything. We are addicted to the machine because we are constantly stimulated. He never shuts down and he never stops.

Many of my clients with sleep issues are so addicted to technology that they have a literal "Fear of Missing Out." This FOMO, as it's called, is a real problem. They become so obsessed with all of the nonsense that they find at their fingertips that they become a slave to it. Technology has officially made them into shells of a person, they no longer know who they are, they have become human robots.

What happened and what can we do to fix it? The ultimate question is: How do we find balance? We aren't all going to sell our earthly possessions and move into a tiny house in the mountains. It would be a life altering experience, but we need to stay a bit more realistic. Balance is an elusive word. We use it often and think of it as something that can never be obtained. But is that true? Are we lying to ourselves before we even explore the truth so that we have an excuse not to commit? Commitment is huge! If we do not commit, we do nothing.

The big question is, how do you find balance between technology and nature? You have to **want** it. It's as simple as that. Do you want that kind of balance? Right now, you might have mixed emotions. You want to connect, but you also want to sit on the couch watching Netflix and catching up on Instagram. Why is that?

When we try something new, we attach a massive amount of fear to it. We are scared out of our minds. We internalize every possible negative scenario and talk ourselves out of even beginning.

When I think about hiking with my father I immediately think of how hardcore he is and I freak out a little. I think, "Oh man, he is going to make me work for it." Nine times out of ten, I have this internal reaction, but guess what? I go hiking anyway. I charge the mountain like a boss. And so can you! The trick is this: if you do something alone, you do what you can handle. If you go with a partner, they push you to achieve more. My dad is my number one fan; he always pushes me to do my best. Despite my internal dialogue, he helps me kill it every time!

Being connected to the outdoors brings us clarity, hope, perseverance, pain, and accomplishment. There is nothing like making a date with nature and seeing it through, she will please us every time!

CHAPTER 11
Unlocking Your Happy Weight

If you get the inside right, the outside will fall into place.

Eckhart Tolle

How does any of this book apply to your weight and health? It has everything to do with everything. You may not have understood this information the first time around, and maybe only bits and pieces stood out, or maybe, it all made sense. You will all have very different experiences with this information. Some of you may think, "I've read this before and none of this is new." For those of you who feel that way, you are seeking an answer that no book can give you. Only your soul can find the answer.

Where Do We Go From Here?

At this point you might be excited, confused, or upset that I didn't teach you how to lose weight. But if weight loss is still the primary concern after all of this, then you, my sweet friend, have missed the point. My hope is that you will miraculously understand that the person you see in the mirror right now is the most amazing person to ever exist. You are beautiful exactly the way you are, and in my eyes, you are simply perfect.

To understand health in the body is to understand the body as a whole. We create unhealthy lifestyles by engaging in negative lifestyle habits and choices.

If you want to make changes in your health, do it. Don't wait. I am the queen of procrastination, but only because I fear what is at the end of the finish line. Writing this book was terrifying, but finishing it and letting others read it is even more of a gut-wrenching feeling. I didn't wait, and I finished it. Like I said previously, change is hard for everyone, but once you start, you did it, you're making things happen. Simply starting the act of change is half the battle.

We may not currently be in the best health state of our life, but that doesn't mean we cannot achieve it. Toxicity and stress are the primary factors in an unhealthy body. Toxicity can be delivered in so many forms. Harmful foods, bad relationships, and negative self-image all contribute. The stress from these is insurmountable for the body and is what causes us to be ultimately unhealthy. I know women that eat perfectly, but are still unhealthy because of the stress they allow themselves to endure on a daily basis. All of this might sound difficult, but it is so worth the shift, change, and exploration. There is a rainbow at the end of every storm. We have exactly what it takes to makes these changes, to become healthier, happier, and to be our best self.

Brilliance And Perfection Are Inside You

You, yes you, have this amazing thing inside of you that the world needs to see. Only you know what it is, and maybe you are still trying to figure what "it" is, but that's okay.

Exploration is what is going to get you to your happy weight.

For me it was moving to a place that fit my wants in life, going back to school, planting roots, removing staple food groups, starting the path of eating clean, moving my body as often as I could, and respecting my mind, body, and soul. Once I found my groove I felt free, beautiful, accomplished, satisfied. Every day I try to live up to my favorite sentiment of all time: "BE SATISFIED."

Once we let go of expectations, accusations, opinions, ideals, boxes, molds, oppression of any kind, we can begin to live in our happy weight and be satisfied.

Your Health Is Your Responsibility

Now is the time to take the bull by the horns and make strides toward your health and wellness goals. Are you healthy? What does healthy mean? What does it look like?

This is what healthy looks like: Sleeping through the night, having consistent and sustainable energy, balanced hormones, mental clarity, balanced emotions, the ability to handle stressful situations without exploding, daily healthy bowel movements, no cravings, no hangry-ness, no blood sugar imbalances, no headaches or migraines, no unnecessary prescribed medications, no need for over the counter drugs, little to no annual sickness or relapses, no toxic relationships, and no use of toxic household chemicals. All of this is possible if you make your health a priority. That is the true meaning of finding your happy weight: making yourself a priority! Will all of this happen overnight? No way! So, don't try to be prefect, no one is! If you can achieve any one of those on the list, you are on your way! You are doing great! Keeping fighting for what makes you happy!

Three Tips To Unlocking Your Happy Weight

Tip 1: Testing

Be very aware of the style of allopathic testing from general practitioners. They are not designed to pick up on the subtle changes in the body, and they can often be very discouraging and inconclusive. Typically, these tests are a gauge for illness or a marker to implement pharmaceutical drugs. You need tests that confirm real time variability with hormones like cortisol, or with nutrients like zinc. I have had so many clients with zinc deficiencies that have derailed their health by making them lose their taste for meat, causing severe iron deficiency, and not producing adequate stomach acid that caused many inflammatory conditions. These tiny fixes can make the world of difference.

Find a legitimate functional medicine physician or naturopathic physician who specializes in genetic, auto immune, salivary hormone, vitamin/mineral, metal toxicity hair analysis, food sensitivity, gut microbiome, cardiovascular, and blood sugar tests.

If you do not have those types of physicians near to you these are amazing "mail in" tests that are changing the game: 23 and Me, Igenix, Everlywell, Labrix, Ubiome, ARLTMA...

These kinds of tests could save your life.

This is where you start to understand how your individual body actually works and what the root cause of your inflammation/health issues might be.

Tip 2: Detoxify Your Home And Life

So many women suffer from exposure to endocrine disrupters. Endocrine disrupters cause issues like estrogen dominance, thyroid deficiency, auto immune flares, cancer, and more. According to a 2012 study conducted by the World Health Organization, endocrine disruptors are described as: "Endocrine disrupting chemicals (EDCs) and potential EDCs are mostly man-made, found in various materials such as pesticides, metals, additives or contaminants in food, and personal care products. EDCs have been suspected to be associated with altered reproductive function in males and females; increased incidence of breast cancer, abnormal growth patterns and neurodevelopmental delays in children, as well as changes in immune function."[1]

Human exposure to EDCs occurs via ingestion of food, dust, and water, via inhalation of gases and particles in the air, and through the skin. EDCs can also be transferred from a pregnant woman to the developing fetus or child through the placenta and breast milk. Pregnant mothers and children are the most vulnerable populations to be affected by developmental exposures, and the effect of exposures to EDCs may not become evident until later in life. Research also shows that it may increase the susceptibility to non-communicable diseases."[2]

These are household chemicals hiding in your shampoo, lotion, perfume, deodorant, hand soap, window cleaner, and candles. They are in any single thing with fragrance or chemicals you can't pronounce. These toxic items can contribute in large ways to your health issues, and it would be in your best interest to throw them away. When looking for replacements of household and body care products look for terms like *gluten free, paraben free, nontoxic, organic, and chemical free.* They could save your life!

Another topic of importance when discussing detoxification, is ridding yourself of toxic personalities, or recalibrating your relationships with others. There may be some people in your life that aren't concerned with you growing as a positive individual. You cannot achieve your balance or happy weight with people that don't believe in you as an individual. These people are disguised as feeders, body-shamers, naysayers, and anyone that makes you feel guilty, shamed, negative, or simply unpleasant after you speak with them. Re-evaluate and recalibrate. Shift your perspective of said relationships and move them into either distant encounters or try your best to gain control over the conversation and use your voice.

For example: Imagine someone makes a negative comment such as, "Are you really going to eat that?" Your rebuttal, in your own, confident voice, can be something like, "Yes I am, is there something bothering you about what it is that I am eating? Am I not allowed to enjoy my food?" Remember, use your voice!

Tip 3: Find A Daily Movement And Self-Care Routine

If you do not make time for yourself and chose to say you are "too busy," you are making excuses not to take care of yourself. Find a daily routine that you like, not one that is forced on you.

If you like to swim, swim. If you like to walk, walk every day. If you like to ride your bike, ride it everywhere. Physical exercise is imperative to being a healthy individual. If you do not sweat, you will trap all of the toxins you accumulate on a daily basis inside of your body and it will create disease. Treat yourself! Hot baths, sauna, reiki, massage, cupping, dry brushing, acupuncture, these are not luxuries!

Most health concerns comes back to you being too stressed. Do you typically stress eat processed foods when you are in a state of disarray? When you think negative thoughts and emotions, did you know you elevate your blood pressure, and can disrupt your digestive tract? There are so many stress induced issues that affect health. If you do not prioritize self-care you will be no better off than you were before. These self-care acts are necessary to achieving your optimal health and wellness. People say these services are "too expensive," but so are the hospital bills you will have to pay when your body decides to give up on you because you have given up on it.

We always make excuses as to why we spend hundreds if not thousands of dollars on beauty products, clothing, or our daily Starbucks, but we refuse to get a once a month massage that could be life altering. Priorities change when we look at what is truly important and see the need to take care of the only body we get.

Resources To Eat Clean And Live Clean

Along with everything you have learned, here is a food and home guide to help you be successful on your path to finding your happy weight.

Foods To Eat

- Fresh organic fruits and vegetables (some people would do best to leave nightshades, such as tomatoes, potatoes, peppers, and eggplants completely out)
- Foods made from scratch

- Grass-fed, raw, and cultured dairy (some people would do best to leave dairy completely out)

- Healthy, organic, and grass-fed cooking fats and oils, including avocado oil, coconut oil, tallow, lard, duck fat, ghee, and butter

- Non-GMO, organic, soaked, and sprouted certified gluten-free grains (some people would do best to leave grains completely out)

- Grass-fed and pasture-raised bone broth

- Raw, fermented, probiotic-rich foods and beverages like sauerkraut, kombucha, and kimchi

Foods To Avoid

- All genetically modified foods

- Foods that give you digestive stress

- Non-organic/conventional produce

- Trigger foods for binging (try to recreate cleaner options)

- Highly processed and denatured foods

- Anything with unpronounceable chemicals

- Foods that keep you up at night or cause weird nightmares

- Toxic oils, like canola, margarine, corn, and vegetable oil

- GMO and uncultured or non-sour wheat products

- Ultra-pasteurized and denatured dairy products

- Farm-raised fish

- Products/recipes that don't only use completely natural and organic ingredients

- Foods with fillers, such as rice starch, soy lecithin, and guar gum

Now is the time to investigate, put yourself out there, ask questions, get answers, and don't stop until you get there. Find your HAPPY WEIGHT!

Bibliography

Wheat Belly by Dr. William Davis
http://www.wheatbellyblog.com
The Wahls Protocol by Dr. Terry Wahls
http://www.terrywahls.com
Grain Brain, Brain Maker by Dr. David Perlmutter
http://www.drperlmutter.com
The Whole Soy Story by Dr. Kaayla Daniel
http://www.drkaayladaniel.com
The GAPS Diet by Dr. Natasha Campbell McBride
http://www.thegapsdiet.com
The Autoimmune Wellness Handbook by Mickey Trescott and Angie Alt
http://www.autoimmune-paleo.com
Nutrition and Physical Degeneration by Dr. Weston A. Price
http://www.westonaprice.org
Pottenger's Cats by Dr. Francis M. Pottenger
Nourishing Traditions by Sally Fallon
http://www.nourishingtraditions.com
Pottenger's Prophecy by Gray Graham

Notes

INTRODUCTION

1. Cynthia Ogden, Ph.D., et al, "Prevalence of Obesity among Adults and Youth: United States, 2011–2014," *Center for Disease Control, NCHS data brief no. 219* (November 2015). Available at: https://www.cdc.gov/nchs/data/databriefs/db219.pdf

CHAPTER 1   HAPPY WEIGHT

1. "Psychological Projection," Available at Wikipedia (accessed on November 29, 2016). Available at: http://en.wikipedia.org/wiki/Psychological_projection

2. "Microbiome," National Human Genome Research Institute (accessed on November 29, 2016). Available at https://www.genome.gov/glossary/index.cfm?id=502&textonly=true

3. International Journal of Obesity (1997) 21, 738-746, Stockton Press.

   Available at (accessed on December 4th, 2016).

http://www.nature.com/ijo/journal/v21/n9/pdf/0800473a.pdf?origin=publication_detail

Chapter 2 The Journey to Happy Weight

Epigraph. Available at http://www.oprah.com/spirit/Oprahs-Experience-with-John-of-God-Oprah-on-Lifes-Journey

1. "Ketogenics," Available at Wikipedia (accessed on December 4, 2016) https://en.wikipedia.org/wiki/Ketogenic_diet

2. Malcolm Gladwell. *Outliers* (New York: Back Bay Books, 2008).

3. Louis Lasagna. *The Hippocratic* Oath (Boston, MA.: Tufts University, 1964).

4. National Center for Health Statistics. Health, United States, 2015: With Special Feature on Racial and Ethnic Health Disparities. Hyattsville, MD. 2016. Available at http://www.cdc.gov/nchs/data/hus/hus15.pdf#079

5. Daniela Drake. "Big Pharma is America's New Mafia," *Daily Beast* (February 21, 2015). Available at: http://www.thedailybeast.com/articles/2015/02/21/big-pharma-is-america-s-new-mafia.html

6. Nourishing Traditions, Sally Fallon, (1999), New Trends Publishing.

7. "Global Cancer Rates Could Increase by 50% to 15 Million by 2020," World Health Organization (accessed on November 29, 2016). Available at: www.who.int/mediacentre/news/releases/2003/pr27/en

8. Weston A. Price. *Nutrition and Physical Degeneration A Comparison of Primitive and Modern Diets and Their Effects* (New York: Paul B. Hoeber, 1939).

9. Nourishing Traditions, Sally Fallon, (1999), New Trends Publishing.

10. "Obesity," MedLine Plus (accessed November 29, 2016). Available at: https://medlineplus.gov/obesity.html

11. Hippocrates , Circa 400 B.C.E.

12. "Has the HCG Diet Been Shown to Be Safe and Effective?" Mayo Clinic (accessed on November 29, 2016). Available at: http://www.mayoclinic.org/ healthy-lifestyle/weight-loss/expert-answers/hcg-diet/ faq-20058164

Chapter 3   Bioindividuality

1. Louise Foxcroft, "Calories and Corsets: A history of dieting over 2,000 years", (Profile Books, London 2011).

2. Sylvester Graham. *Lectures on the Science of Human Life* (Boston, MA.: Marsh, Capen, Lyon, and Webb, 1839).

3. "Body Dysmorphic Disorder," *Diagnostic and Statistical Manual of Mental Disorders DSM-5,* American Psychiatric Association (2013). Available at: http://www.psychiatry-online.org.

4. "Get the Facts about Eating Disorders," National Eating Disorder Association (accessed on November 30, 2016). Available at: http://www.nationaleatingdisorders.org/ get-facts-eating-disorders

5. "Anorexia Nervosa," Ibid. Available at: http://www. psychiatryonline.org

6. Bryan Miller, "How Crash Diets Harm Your Health", (CNN.com 2010).

   Available at http://www.cnn.com/2010/ HEALTH/04/20/crash.diets.harm.health/

7. Chris Iliades, MD, "Hypothyroidism Symptoms in Men" (everydayhealth.com 2013). Available at http:// www.everydayhealth.com/thyroid-conditions/hypothy-roidism-symptoms-in-men.aspx

8.   Leaky gut definition available at http://www.webmd. com/digestive-disorders/features/leaky-gut-syndrome#1

9.   Stephan Bischoff, et al. "Intestinal Permeability—A New Target for Disease Prevention and Therapy," *National Library of Medicine, National Institutes of Health* (2014). Available at: https://www.ncbi.nlm.nih.gov/pmc/articles/ PMC4253991

10.   Digestion Chart commissioned on Fiverr.com in Nov 2015 and designed by Chloezola526

11.   Bryan Walsh. "Eat Butter," *Time* (June 23, 2014).

12.   Terry Wahls. *The Wahls Protocol: A Radical New Way to Treat All Chronic Autoimmune Conditions Using Paleo Principles* (New York: Avery Publishing, 2014).

13.   Nora Gedgaudas. *Primal Body Primal Mind* (2009).

14.   Sir Isaac Newton first presented his three laws of motion in the "Principia Mathematica Philosophiae Naturalis" in 1686. You can see this graphically represented on the NASA website. Available at: https://www.grc.nasa.gov/ www/k-12/airplane/newton3.html

15.   Denise Minger. *Death by Food Pyramid* (Primal Nutrition, 2014),

16.   T. Colin Campbell. *The China Study* (Philadelphia, PA.: BenBella Books, 2005).

17.   Keys, Ancel, C. Aravanis, H. Blackburn, R. Buzina, B.S Djordjevic, A.S. Dontas, F. Fidanza, M.J. Karvonen, N. Kimura, A. Menotti , I. Mohacek , S. Nedeljkovic, V. Puddu, S. Punsar, H.L. Taylor, F.S.P. Van Buchem. Seven countries. A multivariate analysis of death and coronary heart disease. Cambridge: (1980 Harvard University Press).

18.   Why America Is Fatter and Sicker Than Ever, Arthur Agatston, MD, (American Heart Association, July 2012).

19. Francis M. Pottenger, Jr. *Pottenger's Cats: A Study in Nutrition* (Library of Congress, 2012).

20. Cravings chart commissioned on Fiverr.com in Nov 2015 and designed by Chloezola526

21. Poop chart commissioned on Fiverr.com in Nov 2015 and designed by Chloezola526

22. April Khan. "How Much Waste Can the Intestines Hold?" *New Health Advisor* (accessed November 30, 2016). Available at: http://www.newhealthadvisor.com/ How-much-waste-can-the-intestines-hold.html

23. Kellyann Petrucci. *Dr. Kellyann's Bone Broth Diet* (Rodale Books, 2015).

24. Michael Pollan. *Food Rules: An Eater's Manual* (New York: Penguin, 2009).

25. Jane Higdon. "Cruciferous Vegetables," *Linus Pauling Institute* (2005). Available at: http://lpi.oregonstate.edu/

Chapter 4   Vulnerability

Epigraph. Brené Brown, Daring Greatly: How the Courage to Be Vulnerable Transforms the Way We Live, Love, Parent, and Lead (2012)

1. Christiane Northrup. *Women's Bodies, Women's Wisdom: Creating Physical and Emotional Health and Healing* (New York: Bantam Books, 2010).

Chapter 5   Loving Yourself by Releasing Shame and Guilt

Epigraph. Louise L Hay, "You Can Heal Your Life" (Hay House Publishing 1984).

Chapter 6   Breaking Up Is Hard to Do

Epigraph. Maggi Richard is not published, this is her only quote to date.

1. David M. Marquis, DC, DACBN. "How Inflammation Affects Every Aspect of Your Health," (March 7, 2013).

2. Hum Brain Mapp. (Epub 2016 Mar 18).

   Available at https://www.ncbi.nlm.nih.gov/pubmed/26991559

Chapter 7   True Confidence

Epigraph. Norman Vincent Peale, The Power of Positive Thinking (1952).

1. "Women and Hysteria in History of Mental Health." *National Library of Medicine, National Institutes of Health* (October 19, 2012). Available at https://www.ncbi.nlm.nih.gov/pmc/articles/PMC3480686

2. Kim Anami , Available at http://kimanami.com/the-holy-grail-of-the-cervical-orgasm/

3. G Missig, et al. Oxytocin Reduces Background Anxiety in a Fear-Potentiated Startle Paradigm. Neuropsychopharmacology. 2010; 35: 2607–2616.

   K Uvnas-Moberg, et al. Oxytocin, a mediator of anti-stress, well-being, social interaction, growth and healing. Z Psychosom Med Psychother. 2005;51(1):57-80.

4. Daniel F. Kripke,. *The Dark Side of Sleeping Pills* (ebook). Available at: www.darksideofsleepingpills.com

Chapter 9   Selfishness

1. Brené Brown. *Rising Strong* (New York: Random House, 2015).

CHAPTER 10 FIND YOUR TRIBE, FIND YOURSELF

Epigraph. Aristotle 384 BC

1. Marshall Sahlins. "The Origin of Society," *Scientific American,* vol. 203, no. 3, (1960), pp. 76–87.

2. Definition of *wanderlust.* Available at: www.merriam-webster.com/dictionary/wanderlust

3. Nourishing Traditions, Sally Fallon, (1999), New Trends Publishing.

CHAPTER 11 WHERE DO YOU GO FROM HERE?

Epigraph. Eckhart Tolle, The Power of Now: A Guide to Spiritual Enlightenment

"State of the Science of Endocrine Disrupting Chemicals-2012." World Health Organization (2012), WHO library, United Nations Environment Programme.

Available at http://www.who.int/ceh/publications/endocrine/en/

About the Author

Daniele Delle Valle is a certified nutritional therapy practitioner that has spent her life trying to understand how people receive love. Her experience as a nutritional therapist has taken her from clinic, to private practice, to teaching nutrition education in a classroom for young girls, to her passion for writing. After experiencing a countless number of women with negative self-image she felt compelled to write Happy Weight. Her heart knows no bounds and she hopes that this platform will reach a larger audience so that women everywhere can know their worth and love every part of themselves.

66957012R00123

Made in the USA
Charleston, SC
02 February 2017